Simple Mediterranean Cookbook

Tasty Ideas For Good And Healthy Side Dishes And Appetizers

Ben Cooper

Table of contents

Healthy & Quick Energy Bites

Preparation Time: 10 minutes

Cooking Time: 0 minutes

Servings: 20

Ingredients:
2 cups cashew nuts
¼ tsp. cinnamon
1 tsp. lemon zest
4 tbsp. dates, chopped
1/3 cup unsweetened shredded coconut
¾ cup dried apricots

Directions:

1.Line baking tray with parchment paper and set aside.

2.Add all ingredients in a food processor and process until the mixture is crumbly and well combined.

3.Make small balls from mixture and place on a prepared baking tray.

4.Place in refrigerator for 1 hour.

5.Serve and enjoy.

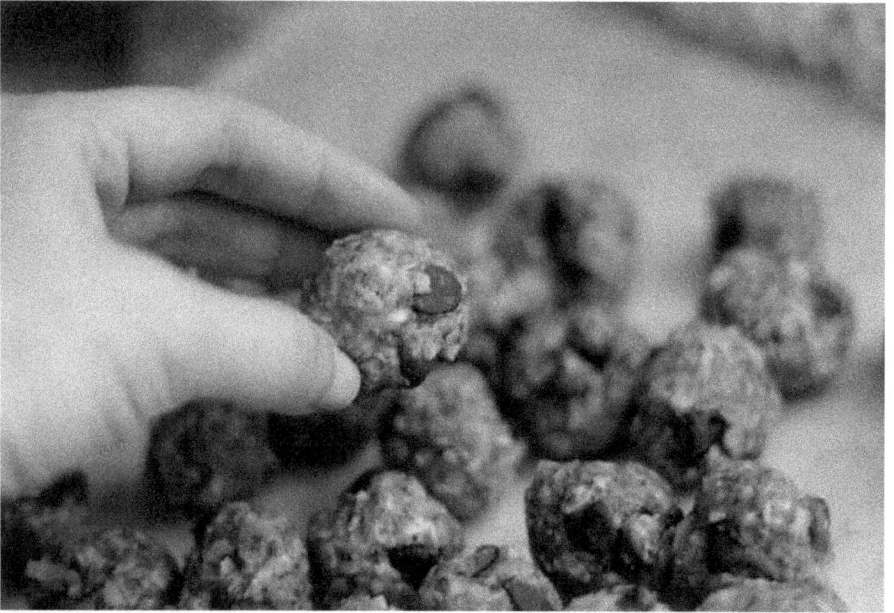

Chicken Wings Platter

Preparation Time: 10 minutes
Cooking Time: 20 minutes
Serves: 4

Ingredients:

2 lb. chicken wings

½ cup tomato sauce

A pinch of salt and black pepper

1 tsp. smoked paprika

1 tbsp. cilantro, chopped
1 tbsp. chives, chopped

Directions:

1.In your instant pot, combine the chicken wings with the sauce and the rest of the ingredients, stir, put the lid on and cook on High for 20 minutes.

2.Release the pressure naturally for 10 minutes, arrange the chicken wings on a platter and serve as an appetizer.

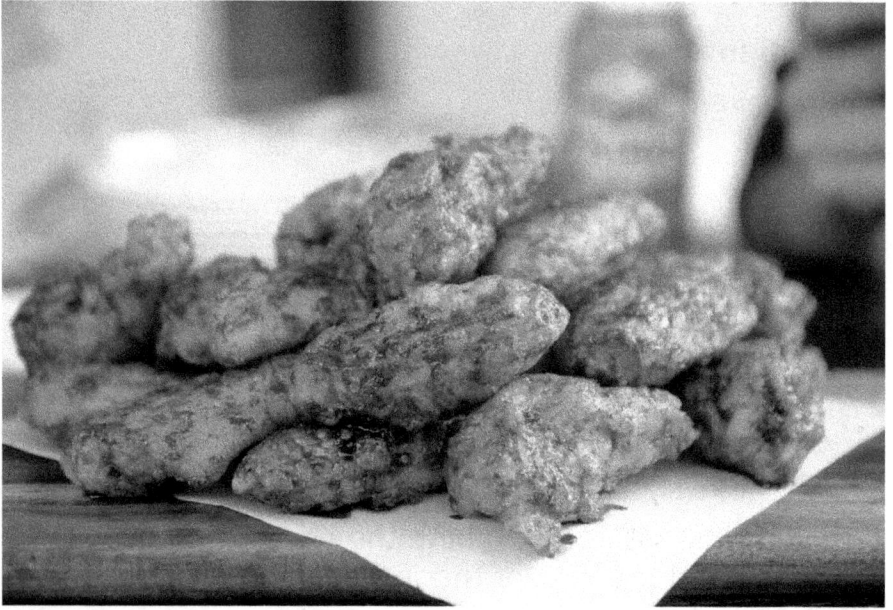

Chocolate Mousse

Preparation Time: 10 minutes
Cooking Time: 6 minutes
Servings: 5

Ingredients:

4 egg yolks
½ tsp. vanilla
½ cup unsweetened almond milk
1 cup whipping cream
¼ cup cocoa powder
¼ cup water
½ cup Swerve
1/8 tsp. salt

Directions:

1.Add egg yolks to a large bowl and whisk until well beaten.

2.In a saucepan, add swerve, cocoa powder, and water and whisk until well combined.

3.Add almond milk and cream to the saucepan and whisk until well mix.

4.Once saucepan mixtures are heated up then turn off the heat.

5.Add vanilla and salt and stir well.

6.Add a tbsp. of chocolate mixture into the eggs and whisk until well combined.

7.Slowly pour remaining chocolate to the eggs and whisk until well combined.

8.Pour batter into the ramekins.

9.Pour 1 ½ cups of water into the instant pot then place a trivet in the pot.

10.Place ramekins on a trivet.

11.Seal pot with lid and select manual and set timer for 6 minutes.

12.Release pressure using quick release method than open the lid.

13.Carefully remove ramekins from the instant pot and let them cool completely.

14.Serve and enjoy.

Veggie Fritters

Preparation Time: 10 minutes

Cooking Time: 10 minutes

Servings: 4

Ingredients:
2 garlic cloves, minced
2 yellow onions, chopped 4 scallions, chopped
2 carrots, grated
2 tsp. cumin, ground
½ tsp. turmeric powder
Salt and black pepper to the taste
¼ tsp. coriander, ground
2 tbsp. parsley, chopped
¼ tsp. lemon juice
½ cup almond flour
2 beets, peeled and grated
2 eggs, whisked
¼ cup tapioca flour
3 tbsp. olive oil

Directions:

1.In a bowl, combine the garlic with the onions, scallions and the rest of the ingredients except the oil, stir well and shape medium patties out of this mix.

2.Heat a pan with the oil over medium-high heat, add the patties, cook for 5 minutes on each side, arrange on a platter and serve.

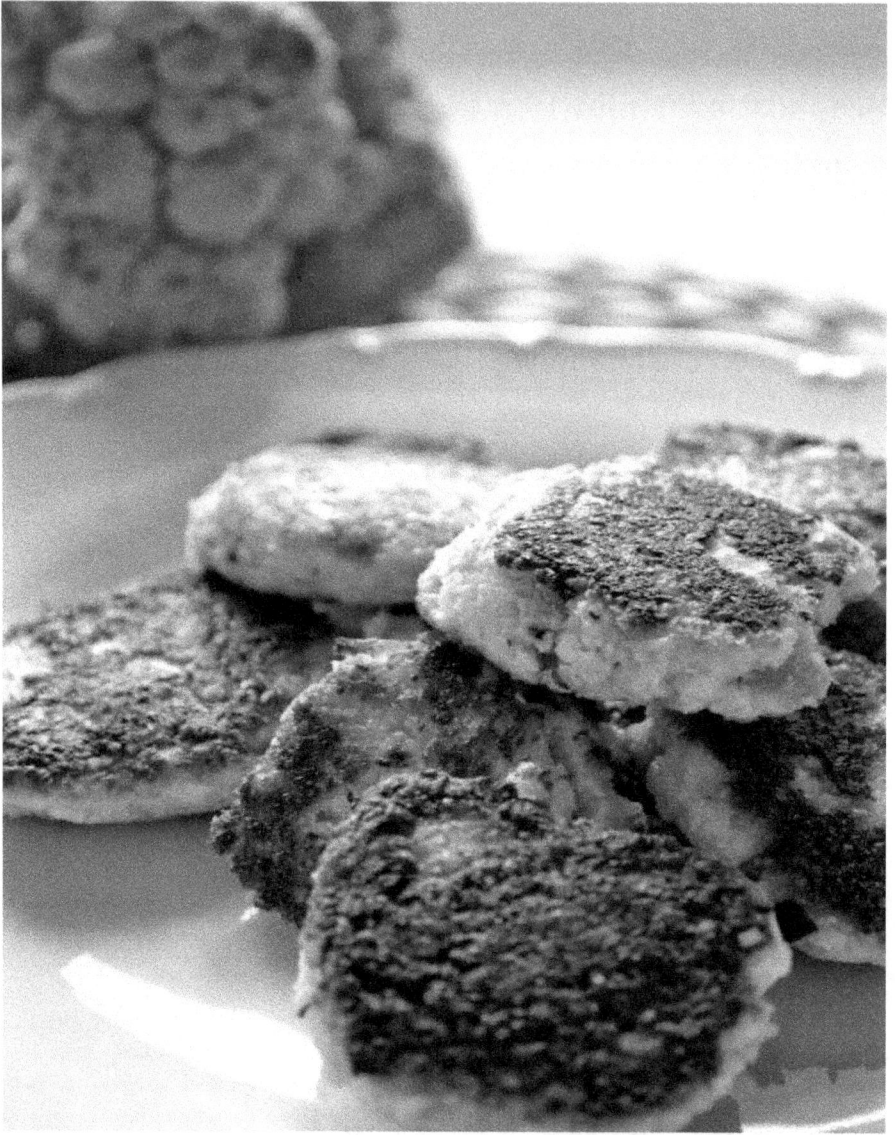

Stuffed Sweet Potato

Preparation Time: 10 minutes
Cooking Time: 40 minutes
Servings: 8

Ingredients:

8 sweet potatoes, pierced with a fork

14 oz. canned chickpeas, drained and rinsed

1 small red bell pepper, chopped

1 tbsp. lemon zest, grated
2 tbsp. lemon juice
3 tbsp. olive oil
1 tsp. garlic, minced
1 tbsp. oregano, chopped
2 tbsp. parsley, chopped
A pinch of salt and black pepper
1 avocado, peeled, pitted and mashed
¼ cup water
¼ cup tahini paste

Directions:

1.Arrange the potatoes on a baking sheet lined with parchment paper, bake them at 400°F for 40 minutes, cool them down and cut a slit down the middle in each.

2.In a bowl, combine the chickpeas with the bell pepper, lemon zest, half of the lemon juice, half of the oil, half of the garlic, oregano, half of the parsley, salt and pepper, toss and stuff the potatoes with this mix.

3.In another bowl, mix the avocado with the water, tahini, the rest of the lemon juice, oil, garlic and parsley, whisk well and spread over the potatoes.

4.Serve cold for breakfast.

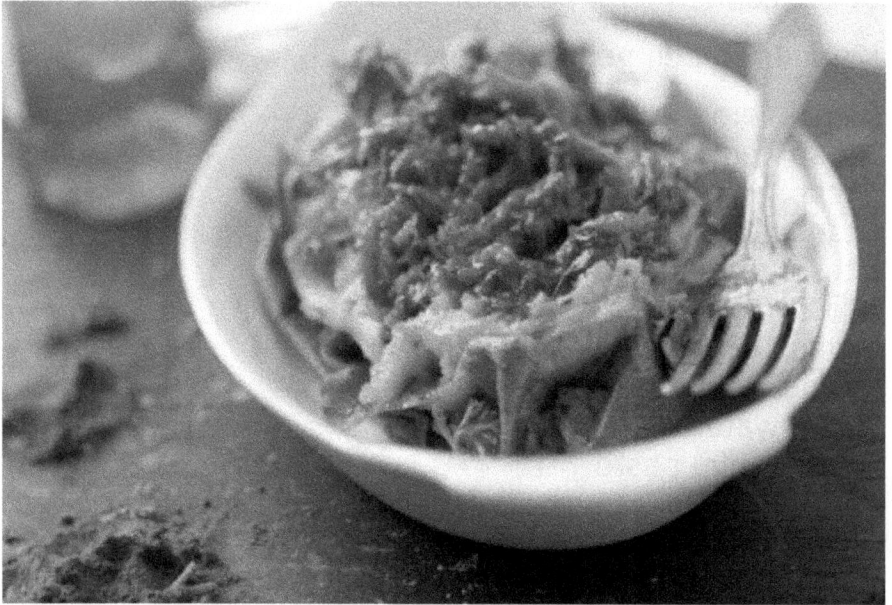

Rosemary Bulgur Appetizer

Preparation Time: 25 minutes

Cooking Time: 0 minutes

Servings: 6

Ingredients:
½ cup couscous 2 tbsp. olive oil
1 ¾ cup onions, chopped
2 cups vegetable broth
1 cup bulgur
1 tbsp. chives, chopped
1 tbsp. parsley, chopped
¼ tsp. rosemary, chopped

Directions:

1.Over medium stove flame; heat the oil in a skillet or saucepan (preferably medium size).

2.Sauté the onions until softened and translucent, stir in between.

3.Add the bulgur and 1 ½ cups vegetable broth; simmer the mixture until the bulgur is tender.

4.Remove it from the heat and fluff with a fork.

5.In another skillet or saucepan, heat the remaining vegetable broth and simmer. Add the oil and couscous. Stir and cook this until your couscous is tender. Fluff it with a fork.

6.In a mixing bowl, combine the bulgur and couscous. Add the rosemary, chives and parsley on top. Season it with black pepper and salt.

7.Serve as an appetizer or light meal.

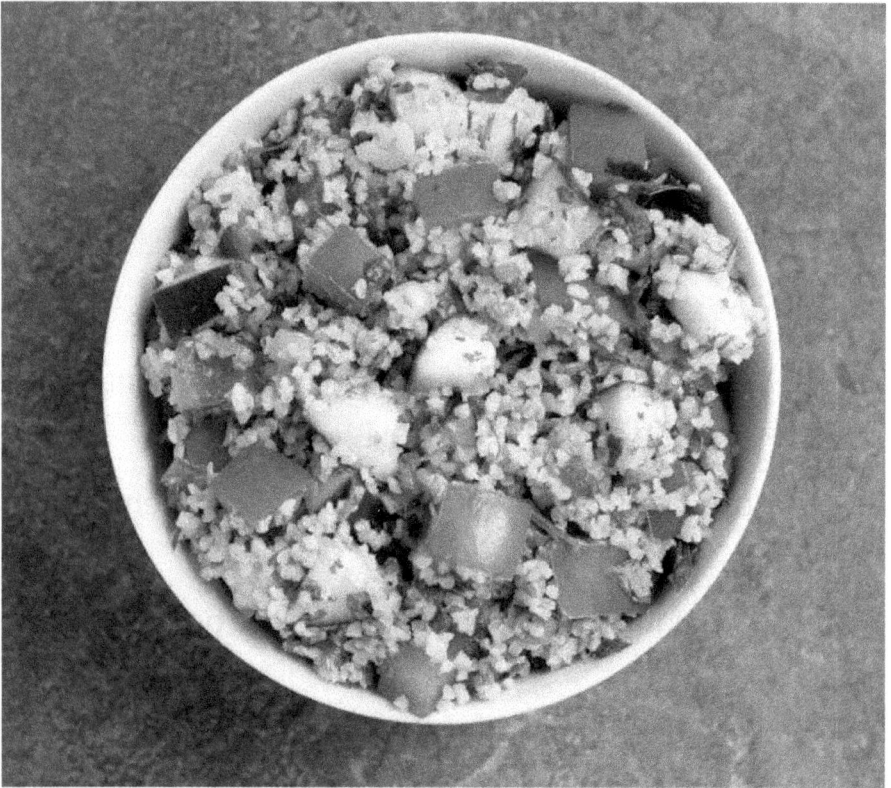

Cauliflower Fritters

Preparation Time: 10 minutes
Cooking Time: 50 minutes
Servings: 4

Ingredients:

30 oz. canned chickpeas, drained and rinsed
2 and ½ tbsp. olive oil
1 small yellow onion, chopped
2 cups cauliflower florets chopped
2 tbsp. garlic, minced
A pinch of salt and black pepper

Directions:

1.Spread half of the chickpeas on a baking sheet lined with parchment pepper, add 1 tbsp. oil, season with salt and pepper, toss and bake at 400°F for 30 minutes.

2.Transfer the chickpeas to a food processor, pulse well and put the mix into a bowl.

3.Heat a pan with the ½ tbsp. oil over medium-high heat, add the garlic and the onion and sauté for 3 minutes.

4.Add the cauliflower, cook for 6 minutes more, transfer this to a blender, add the rest of the chickpeas, pulse, pour over the crispy chickpeas mix from the bowl, stir and shape medium patties out of this mix.

5.Heat a pan with the rest of the oil over medium-high heat, add the patties, cook them for 3 minutes on each side, and serve breakfast.

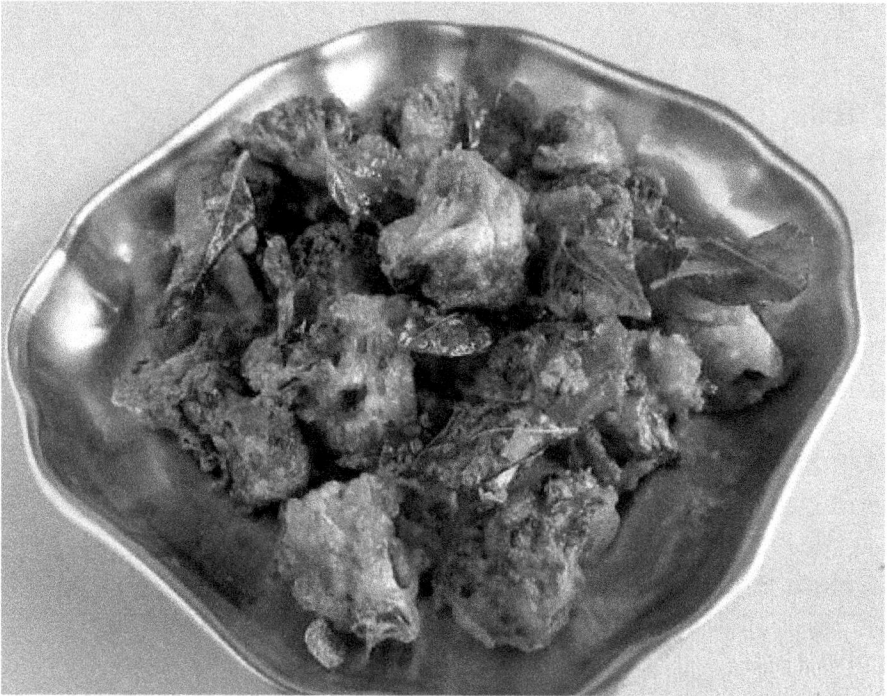

Mediterranean Chickpea Snack

Preparation Time: 30 minutes

Cooking Time: 0 minutes

Servings: 2

Ingredients:

½ tsp. garlic powder
1 can (10 oz.) chickpeas, rinsed and drained
½ tsp. dried basil
1 tsp. extra-virgin olive oil
¼ tsp. sea salt
1 tsp. Nutritional Yeast
¼ tsp. red pepper flakes

Directions:

1.Preheat the oven to 450°F. Line a baking pan with a parchment paper. Grease it with some refined coconut oil or avocado oil (You can also use cooking spray)

2.Combine the chickpeas, seasonings, and oil in a mixing bowl.

3.Arrange the chickpeas in the pan. Roast the chickpeas for about 10 minutes. Toss and keep roasting for 10 more minutes.

4.Serve warm.

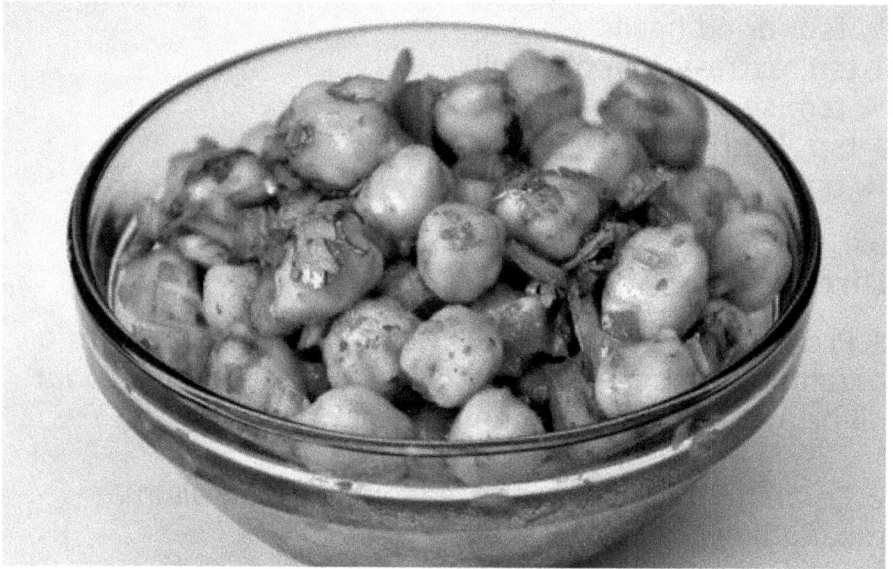

Pita Wedges with Almond Bean Dip

Preparation Time: 10 minutes
Cooking Time: 5 minutes
Servings: 5

Ingredients:
8 oz. beet, cubed
5 garlic cloves, peeled
¼ cup almond, slivered
15 ½ oz. garbanzo beans
¾ cup extra-virgin olive oil
1 ½ tbsp. red wine vinegar
Whole-wheat pita wedges to serve

Directions:

1.In a saucepan or deep skillet, boil the beet in sufficient water quantity until it is tender. Drain, peel, cut in cubes and blend in a food processor.

2.Add the garbanzo beans, almonds, oil, and garlic and blend everything well until smooth. Add the red wine and blend for one more minute.

3.Season with black pepper and salt. Chill in the refrigerator. Serve with pita wedges.

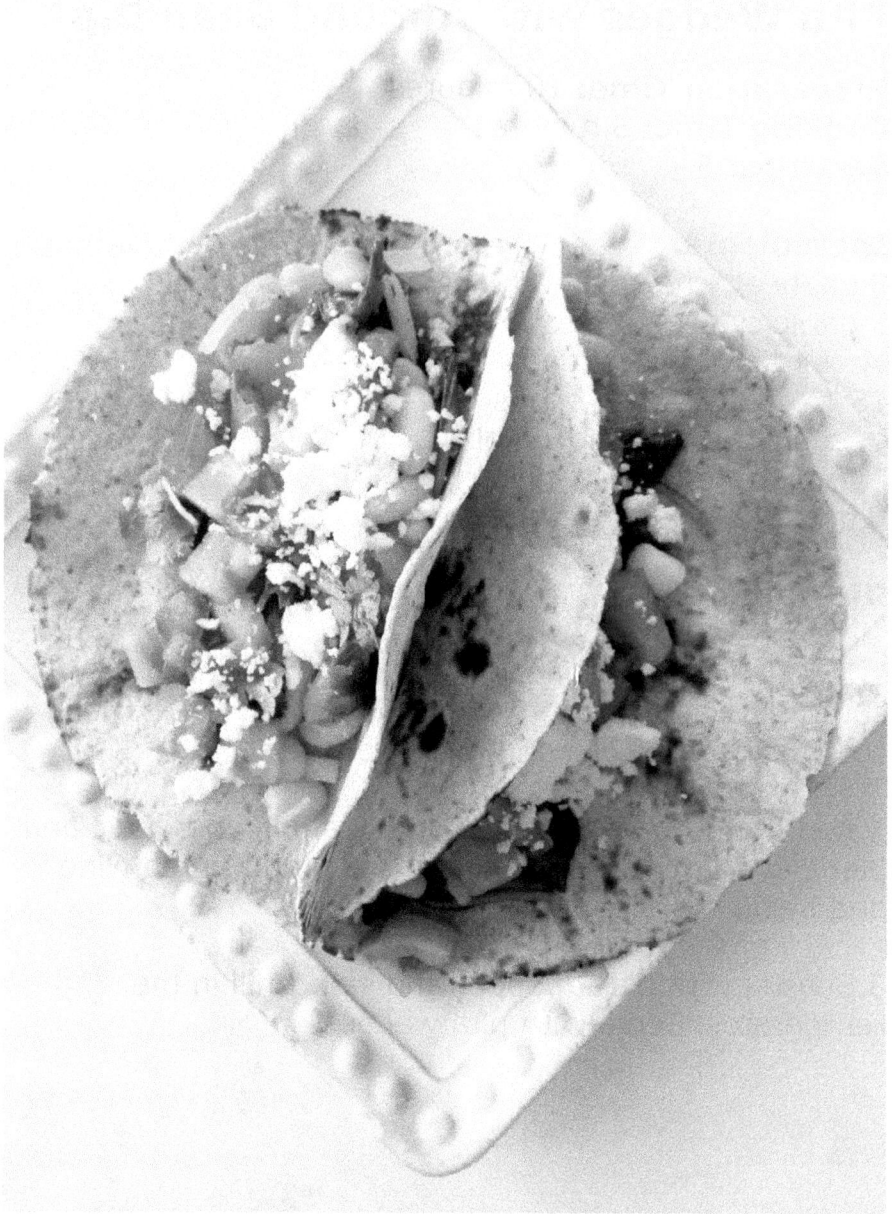

Ginger Antipasti

Preparation Time: 10 minutes
Cooking Time: 0 minutes
Servings: 6

Ingredients:

1 tsp. ginger powder
1 cup fresh parsley, chopped
1 tbsp. apple cider vinegar
3 tbsp. avocado oil
2 oz celery stalk, chopped

Directions:

1.Mix all ingredients in the bowl and leave for 5 minutes in the fridge.

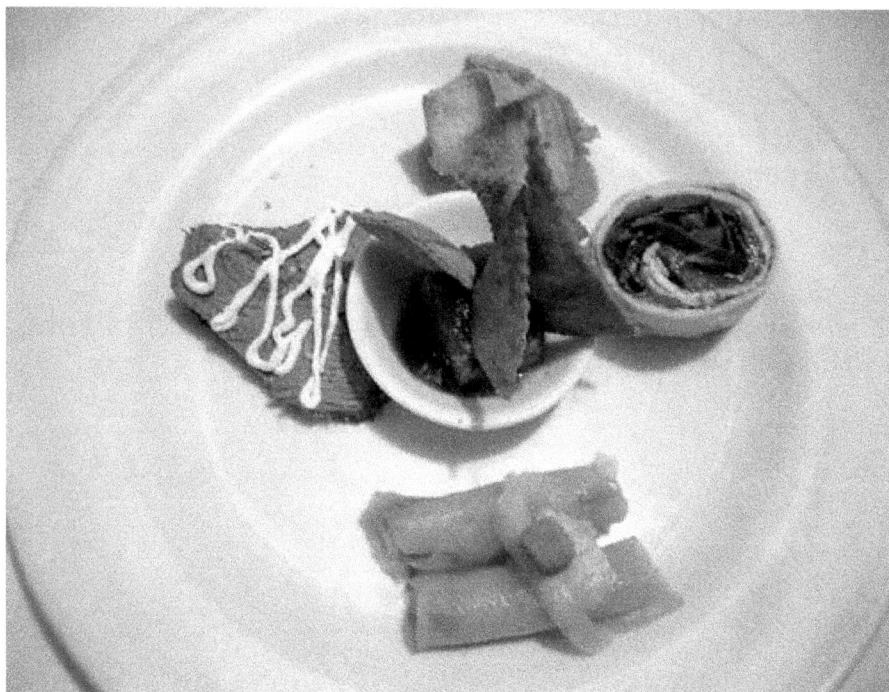

Mediterranean Chickpea Spread

Preparation Time: 8 minutes
Cooking Time: 5 minutes
Servings: 2

Ingredients:

2 cups chickpeas (canned or pre-soaked and cooked)
2 tbsp. lemon juice
1/2 tsp. cumin
2 cloves garlic, minced
4 tsp. olive oil
Salt to taste
Ground cinnamon (optional)

Directions:

1.In a mixing bowl, add the chickpeas; mash thoroughly using a fork (you can also use a blender).

2.Add the olive oil, garlic and lemon juice. Combine well; top with some cinnamon.

3.Serve with vegetable sticks, whole-wheat crackers, or whole-wheat pita wedges.

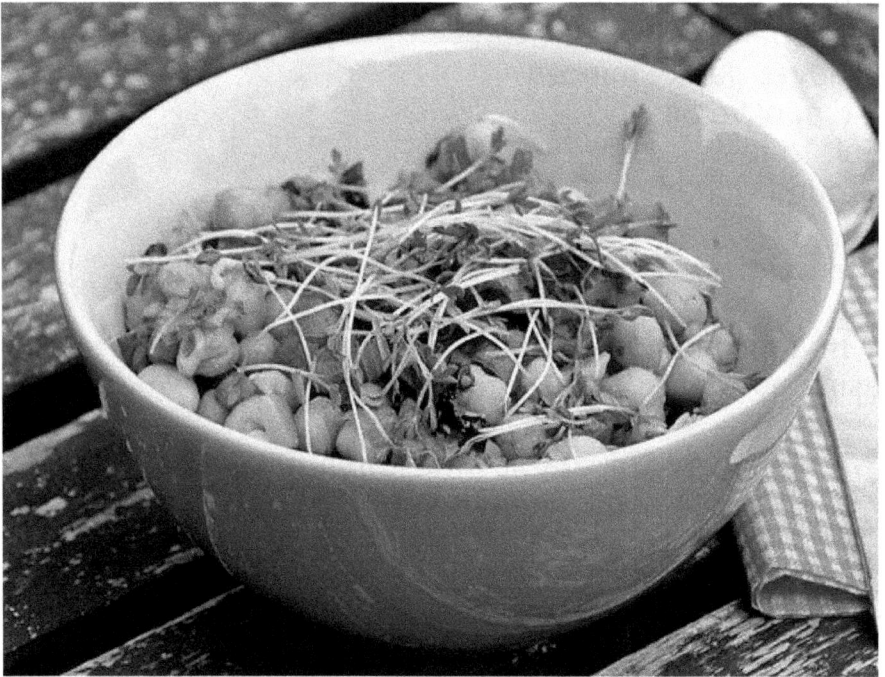

Scallions Dip

Preparation Time: 5 minutes
Cooking Time: 15 minutes
Servings: 4

Ingredients:

1 cup spinach, chopped
2 oz scallions, chopped
¼ cup plain yogurt
¼ tsp. chili powder
1 tsp. olive oil

Directions:

1.Melt the olive oil in the saucepan.

2.Add spinach and scallions.

3.Saute the greens for 10 minutes.

4.Then add chili powder and plain yogurt. Stir well and cook it for 5 minutes more.

5.Then blend the mixture with the help of the immersion blender.

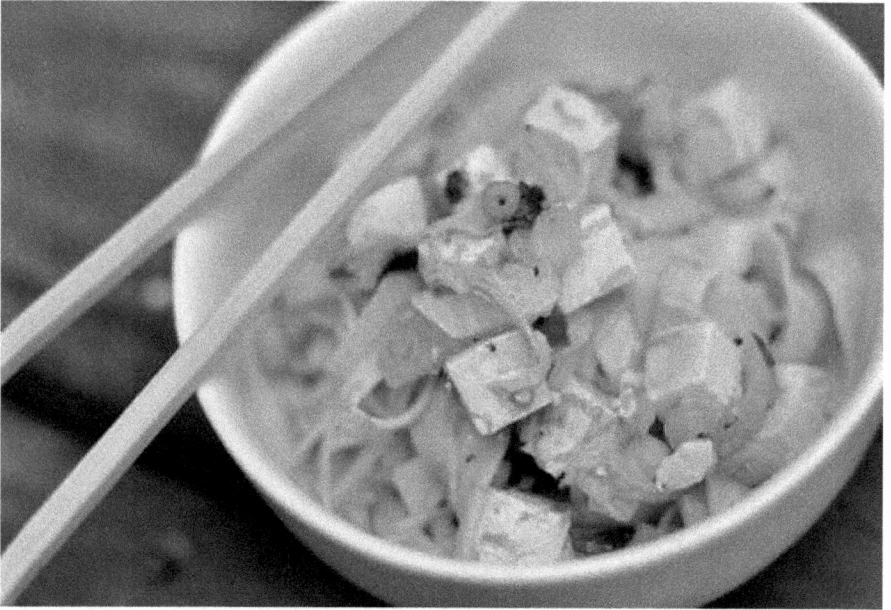

Dill Tapas

Preparation Time: 5 minutes

Cooking Time: 0 minutes

Servings: 8

Ingredients:

½ tsp. garlic powder 2 cups plain yogurt
½ cup dill, chopped
¼ tsp. ground black pepper
2 pecans, chopped
2 tbsp. lemon juice

Directions:

1.Put all ingredients in the bowl and stir well with the help of the spoon.

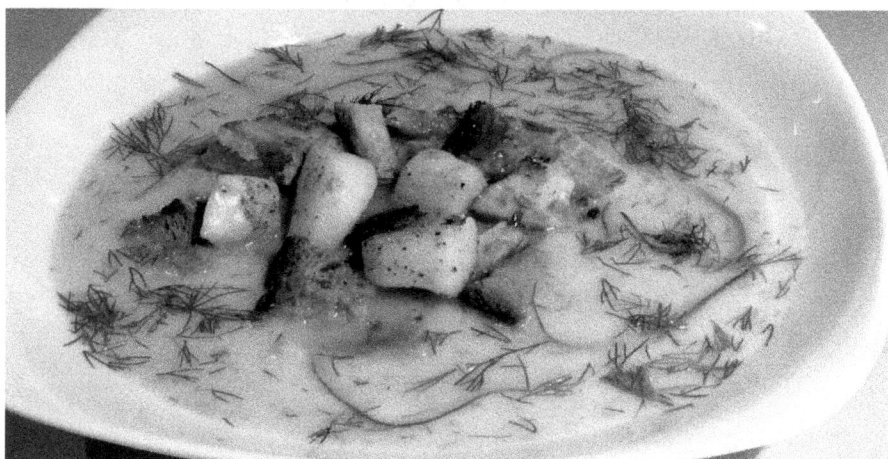

Sour Cream Dip

Preparation Time: 10 minutes
Cooking Time: 0 minutes
Servings: 8

Ingredients:
4 oz yogurt
¼ tsp. chili flakes
¼ tsp. salt
2 avocados, peeled, pitted
1 tsp. olive oil
½ tsp. lemon juice
2 tbsp. fresh parsley, chopped

Directions:

1.Put all ingredients in the blender and blend until smooth.

2.Store the dip in the closed vessel in the fridge for up to 5 days.

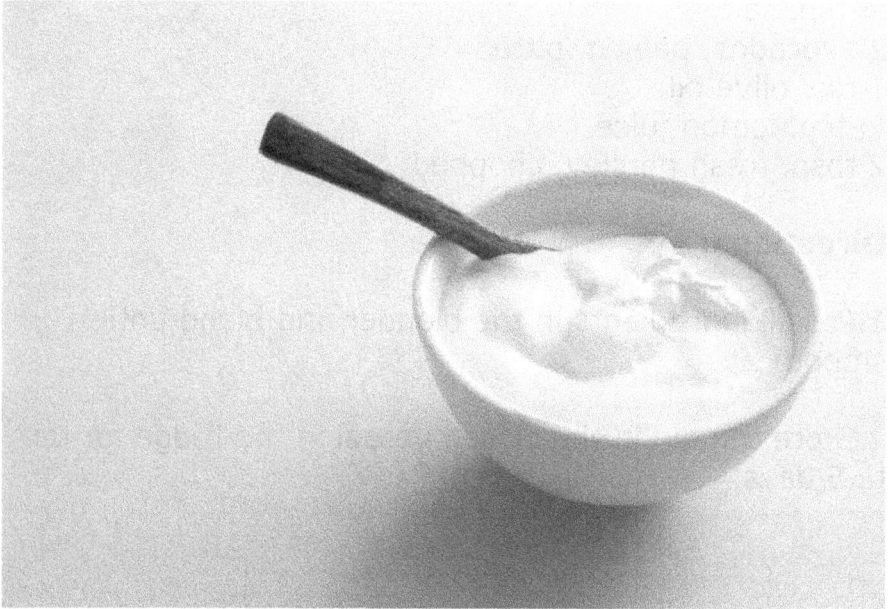

Arugula Antipasti

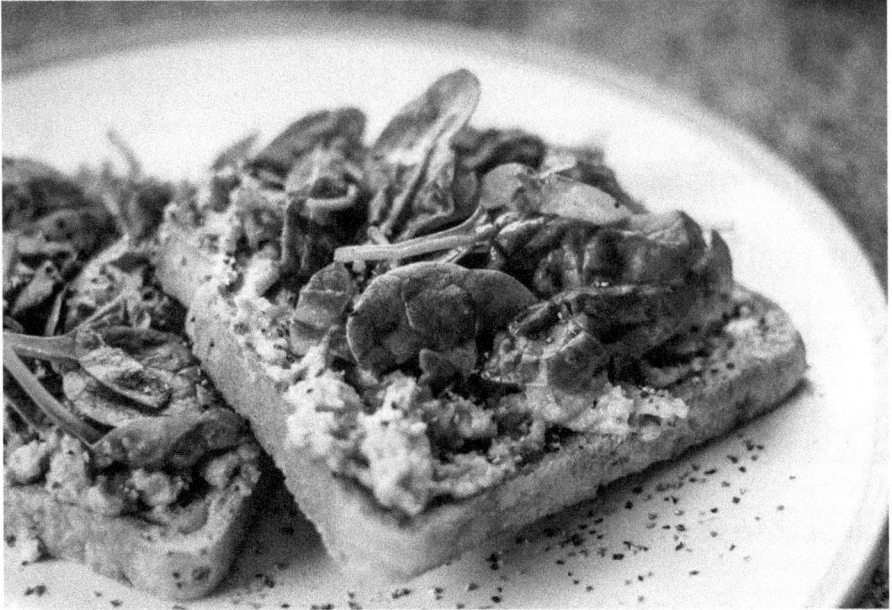

Preparation Time: 5 minutes
Cooking Time: 0 minutes
Servings: 8

Ingredients:

2 oz chives, chopped
1 cup arugula, chopped
2 cups chickpeas, canned
1 jalapeno pepper, chopped 1 tbsp. avocado oil
1 tsp. lemon juice

Directions:

1.Put all ingredients in the bowl and stir well.

Goat Cheese Dip

Preparation Time: 10 minutes
Cooking Time: 8 minutes
Servings: 4

Ingredients:

3 oz goats cheese, soft
2 oz plain yogurt
2 oz chives, chopped
1 tbsp. lemon juice
¼ tsp. ground black pepper
2 bell peppers

Directions:

1Grill the bell peppers for 3-4 minutes per side.

2.Then peel the peppers and remove seeds.

3.Then put bell peppers in the blender.

4.Add all remaining ingredients, blend them well and transfer in the ramekins.

Mozzarella Dip

Preparation Time: 10 minutes
Cooking Time: 20 minutes
Servings: 10

Ingredients:

1-lb. artichoke hearts, diced
¾ cup spinach, chopped
1 cup mozzarella cheese, grated
1 tsp. Italian seasonings
½ tsp. garlic powder
¼ cup organic almond milk

Directions:

1.Put all ingredients in the saucepan, stir well, and close the lid.

2.Saute the meal on low heat for 20 minutes. Stir it from time to time.

3.Then chill the dip well.

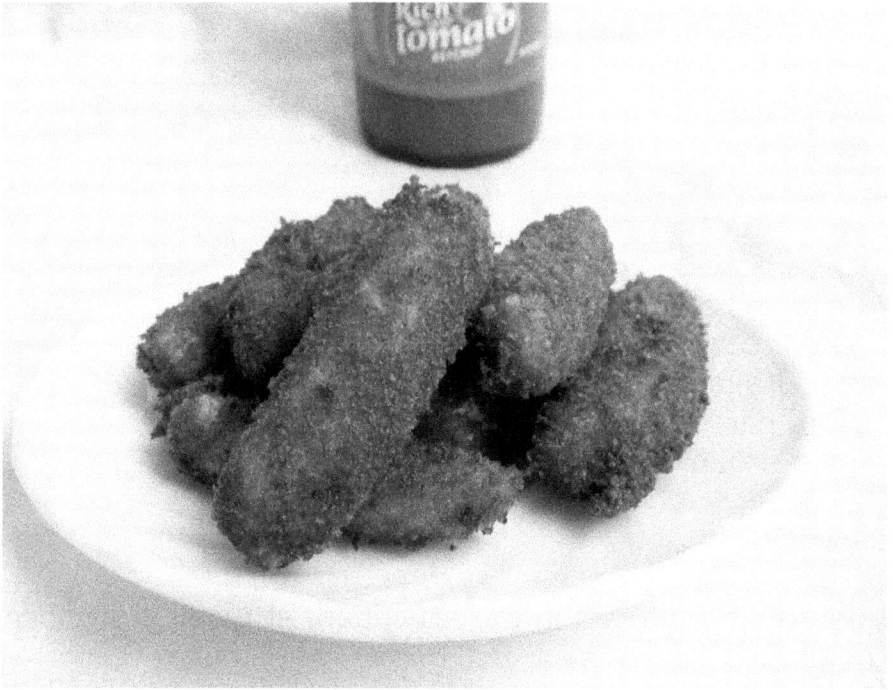

Cheese Spread

Preparation Time: 10 minutes
Cooking Time: 8 minutes
Servings: 6

Ingredients:

½ cup cream cheese 1 pickle, grated
1 oz fresh dill, chopped
¼ tsp. ground paprika

Directions:

1.Carefully mix cream cheese with dill and ground paprika.

2.Then add a grated pickle and gently mix the spread.

Prosciutto Beans

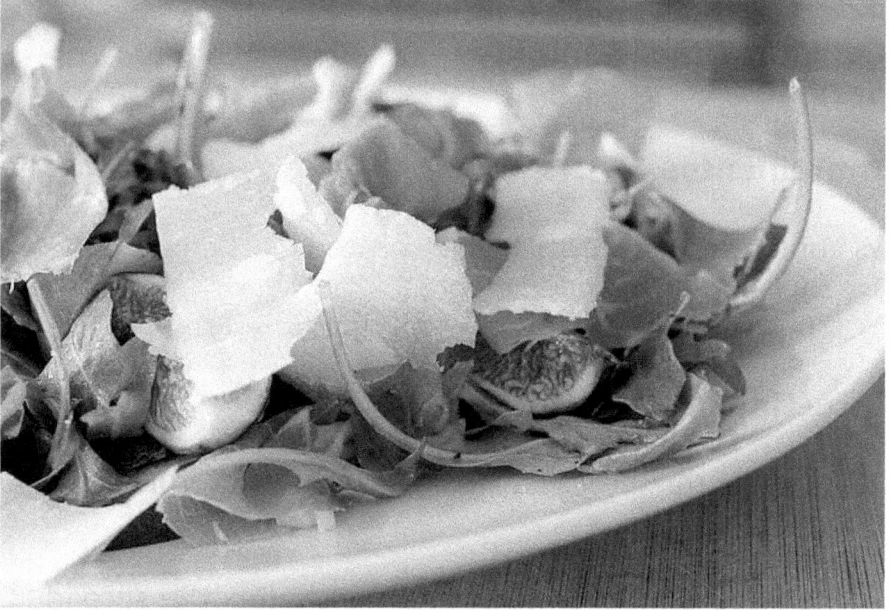

Preparation Time: 10 minutes
Cooking Time: 0 minutes
Servings: 8

Ingredients:
2 cups canned cannellini beans, drained 1 tbsp.
scallions, diced
3 tbsp. olive oil
¼ tsp. chili flakes
1 tbsp. lemon juice
3 oz beef, chopped, cooked

Directions:

1.Put all ingredients in the bowl and stir well.

Carrot Chips

Preparation Time: 5 minutes
Cooking Time: 10 minutes
Servings: 6

Ingredients:
2 carrots, thinly sliced
1 tsp. salt
1 tsp. olive oil
Directions:

1.Line the baking tray with baking paper.

2.Then arrange the sliced carrot in one layer.

3.Sprinkle the vegetables with olive oil and salt.

4.Bake the carrot chips for 10 minutes or until the vegetables are crunchy.

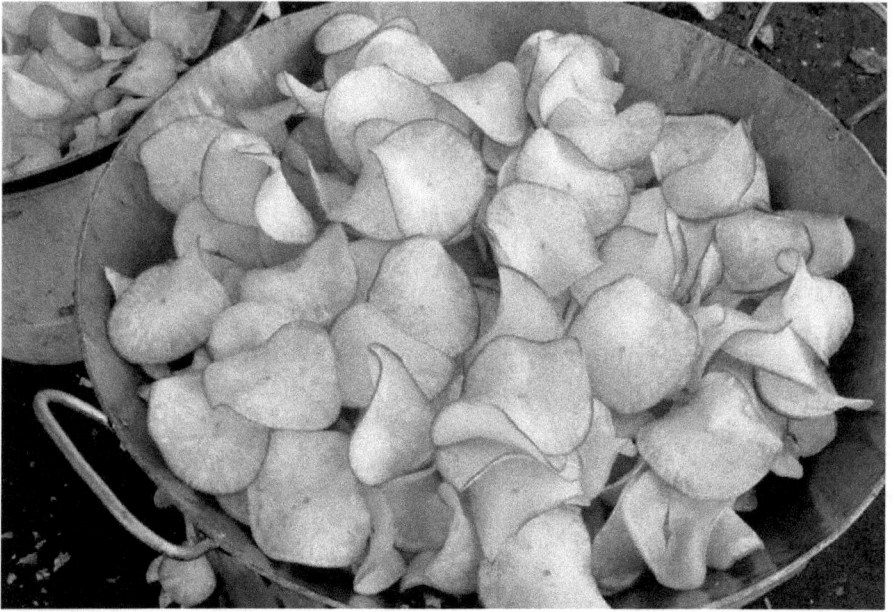

Antipasti Salad

Preparation Time: 10 minutes
Cooking Time: 0 minutes
Servings: 4

Ingredients:

½ cup green olives, pitted and sliced
1 cucumber, spiralized
1 cup cherry tomatoes, halved 4 oz Feta cheese, crumbled
2 tbsp. olive oil

Directions:
1.Put green olives, spiralized cucumber, and cherry tomatoes in the bowl.

2.Add olive oil and stir well.

3.Then top the salad with Feta.

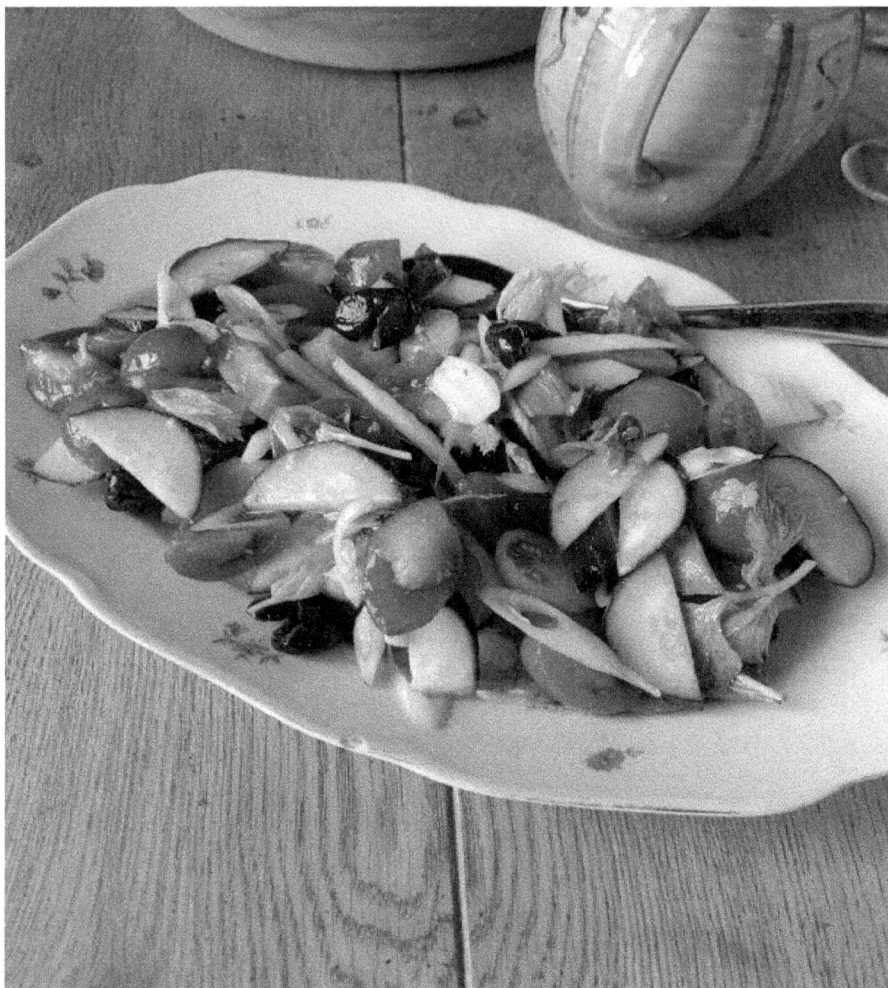

Black Olives Spread

Preparation Time: 10 minutes
Cooking Time: 0 minutes
Servings: 10

Ingredients:
3 cups black olives, pitted
½ cup chickpeas, canned 1 tsp. Italian seasonings 3 tbsp. sunflower oil
½ tsp. ground black pepper

Directions:

1.Put all ingredients in the blender and blend until smooth.

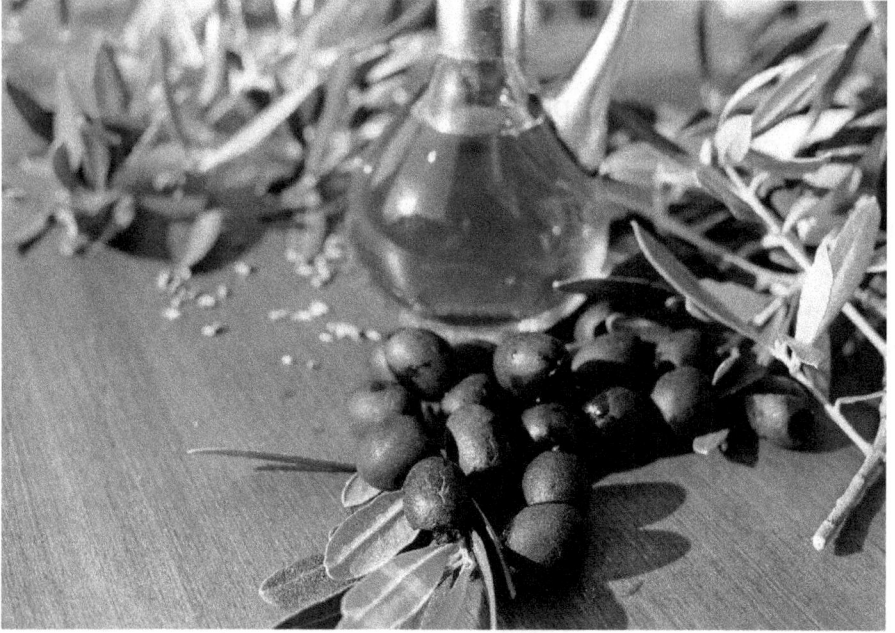

Bell Pepper Antipasti

Preparation Time: 10 minutes
Cooking Time: 4 minutes
Servings: 6

Ingredients:
5 bell peppers
1 tbsp. olive oil
3 tbsp. avocado oil
½ tsp. salt
2 garlic cloves, minced
3 tbsp. fresh cilantro, chopped

Directions:

1.Pierce the bell peppers with the help of a knife and sprinkle with olive oil.

2.Grill the vegetables at 400F for 2 minutes per side.

3.Then peel them and remove seeds.

4.Put the grilled bell peppers in the blender and add all remaining ingredients.

5.Blend the mixture well.

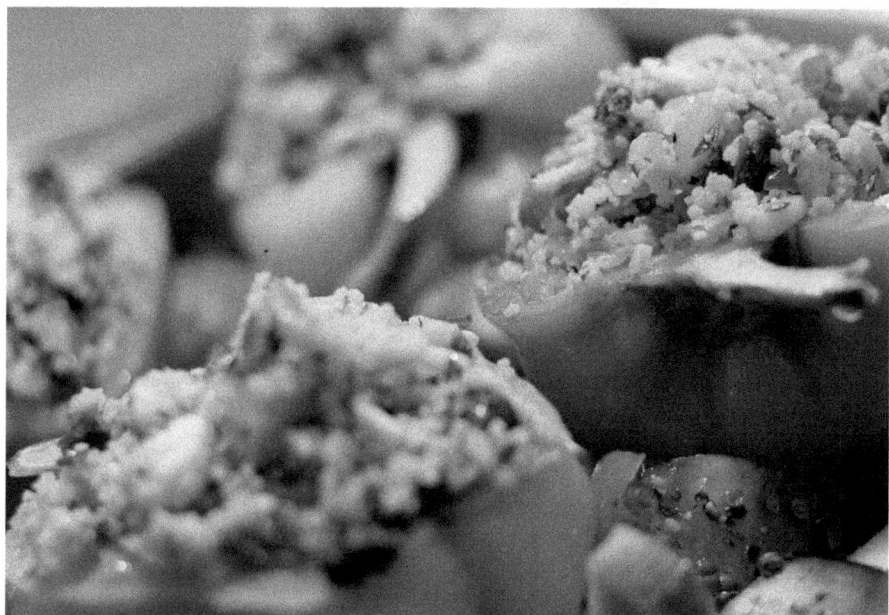

Hummus Rings

Preparation Time: 10 minutes
Cooking Time: 0 minutes
Servings: 4

Ingredients:

½ cup hummus
2 cucumbers

Directions:

1.Roughly slice the cucumbers and remove the cucumber flesh.

2.Then fill every cucumber ring with hummus.

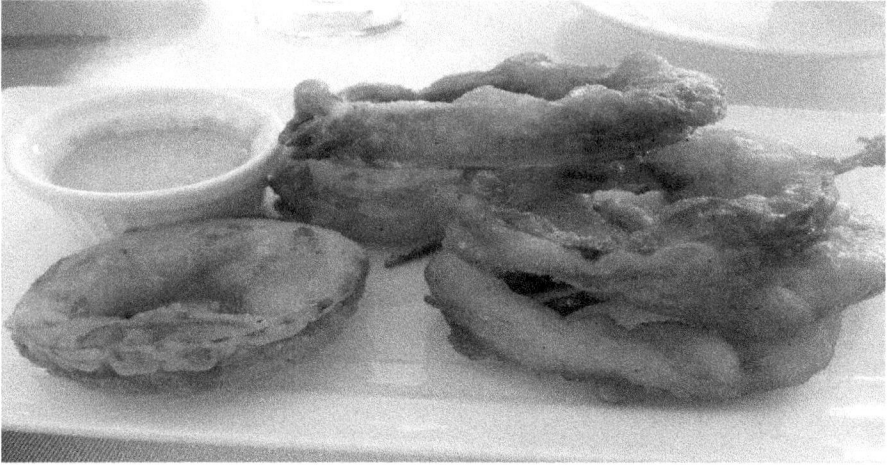

Fish Strips

Preparation Time: 10 minutes
Cooking Time: 0 minutes
Servings: 4

Ingredients:

1 cucumber, sliced
1 tsp. apple cider vinegar
2 tbsp. plain yogurt
1 tsp. dried dill
3 oz salmon, smoked, sliced

 Directions:

1.Arrange the sliced cucumber in the plate in one layer.

2.Then sprinkle them with apple cider vinegar, plain yogurt, and dried dill.

3.Then top the cucumbers with sliced salmon.

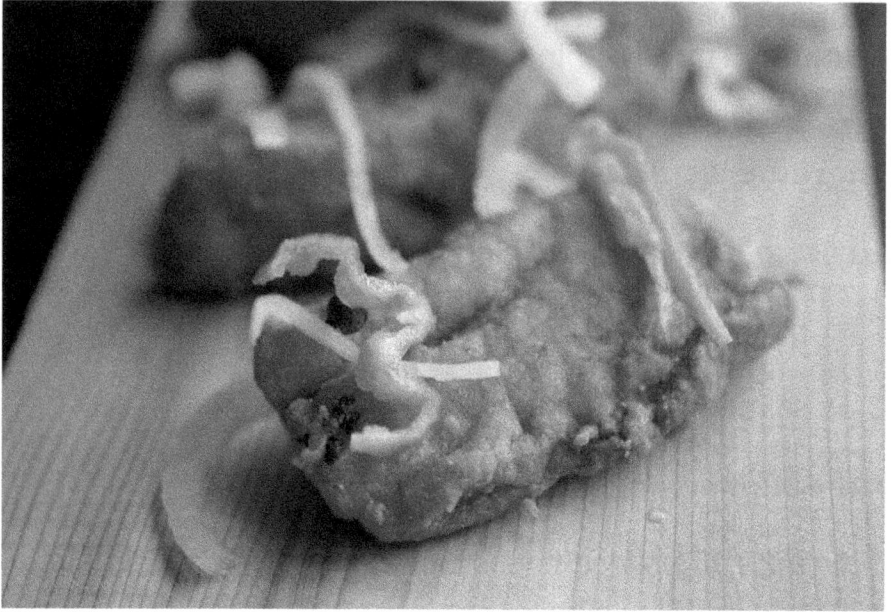

Vegetable Balls

Preparation Time: 10 minutes
Cooking Time: 5 minutes
Servings: 8

Ingredients:
2 eggplants, grilled
2 tbsp. olive oil
1 garlic clove, minced
1 egg, beaten
½ cup oatmeal, ground
½ tsp. ground black pepper
2 oz Parmesan, grated

Directions:

1.Blend the eggplants until smooth.

2.Then mix up blended eggplants with garlic, egg, oatmeal, ground black pepper, and Parmesan.

3.Make the small balls.

4.Heat the skillet with olive oil and put the eggplant balls inside.

5.Roast them for on high heat for 1 minute per side.

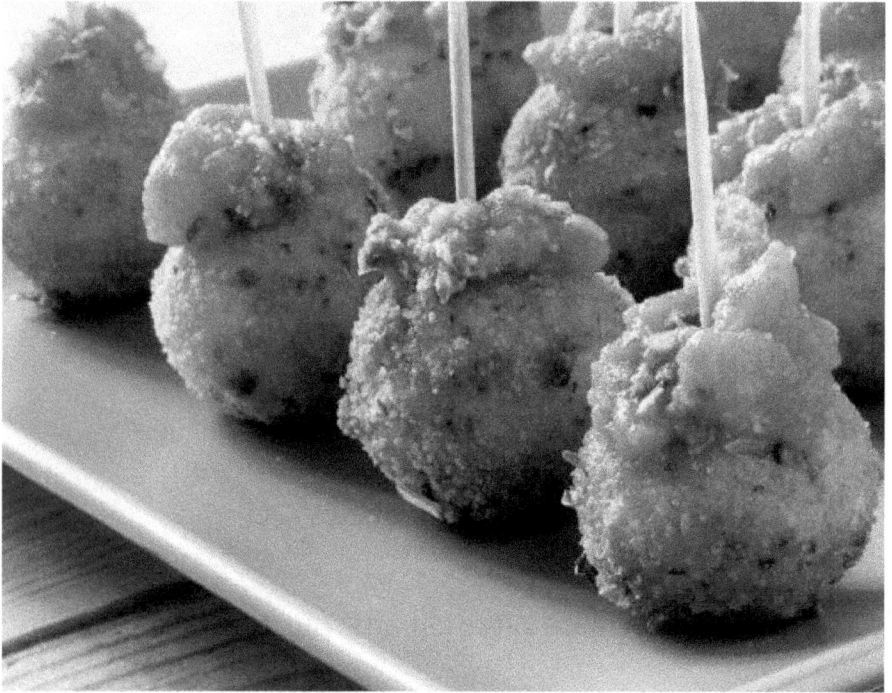

Italian Style Eggplant Chips

Preparation Time: 10 minutes
Cooking Time: 5 minutes
Servings: 10

Ingredients:

2 eggplants, thinly sliced
1 tsp. ground black pepper
1 tsp. Italian seasonings
1 tbsp. olive oil

Directions:

1.Rub the eggplant sliced with ground black pepper and Italian seasonings.

2.Then sprinkle the vegetable sliced with olive oil.

3.Grill the eggplant sliced for 2 minutes per side at 400F or until the vegetables are crunchy.

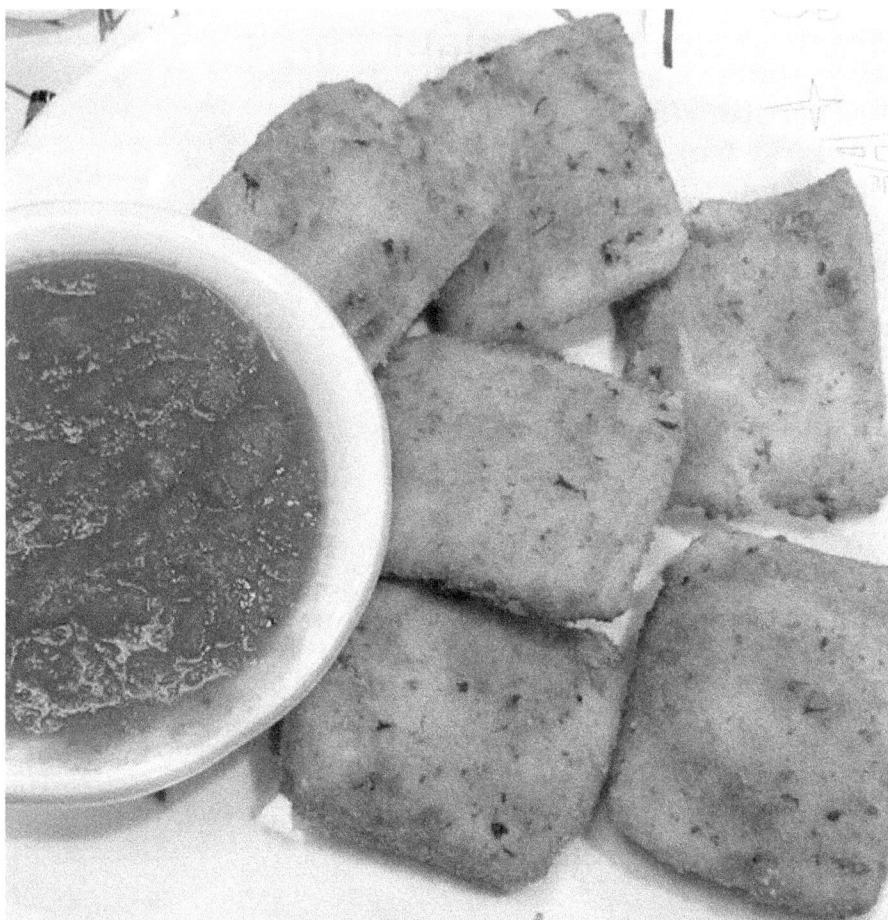

Lentil Dip

Preparation Time: 10 minutes
Cooking Time: 0 minutes
Servings: 7

Ingredients:
1 cup green lentils, cooked
1 tbsp. apple cider vinegar
1 tomato, chopped
1 tsp. olive oil
2 oz Parmesan, grated

Directions:

1.Mix up all ingredients in the bowl and blend gently
with the help of the immersion blender.

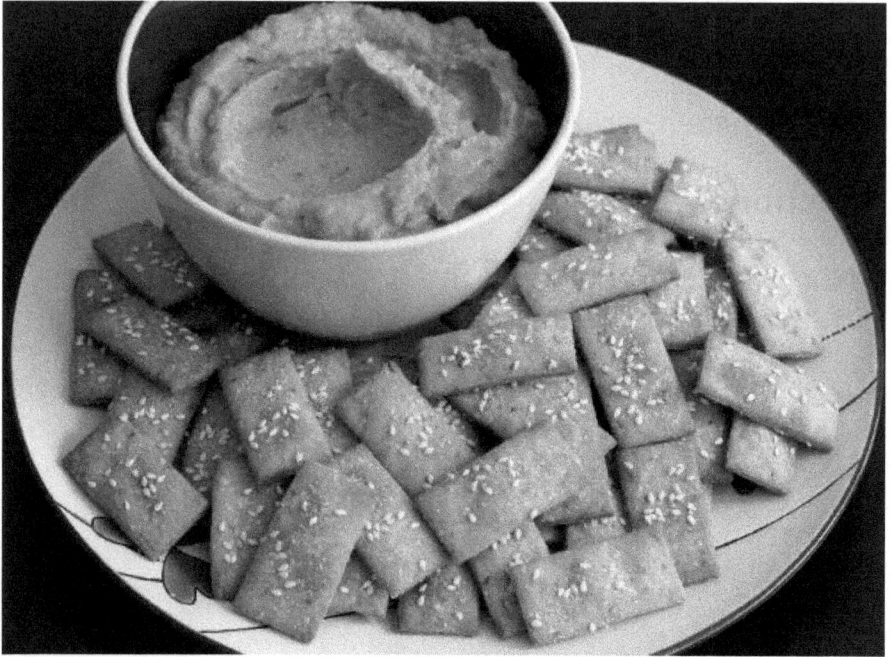

Overnight Oats

Preparation time: 7 minutes
Cooking time: 0 minute
Servings: 2

Ingredients:

1.5 cups Rolled Oats
1 cup Tinned coconut milk
1.5 cup Almond Milk
2 tbsp Chia Seeds
½ tsp Ground Cinnamon

Directions:

1.Blend all the ingredients.

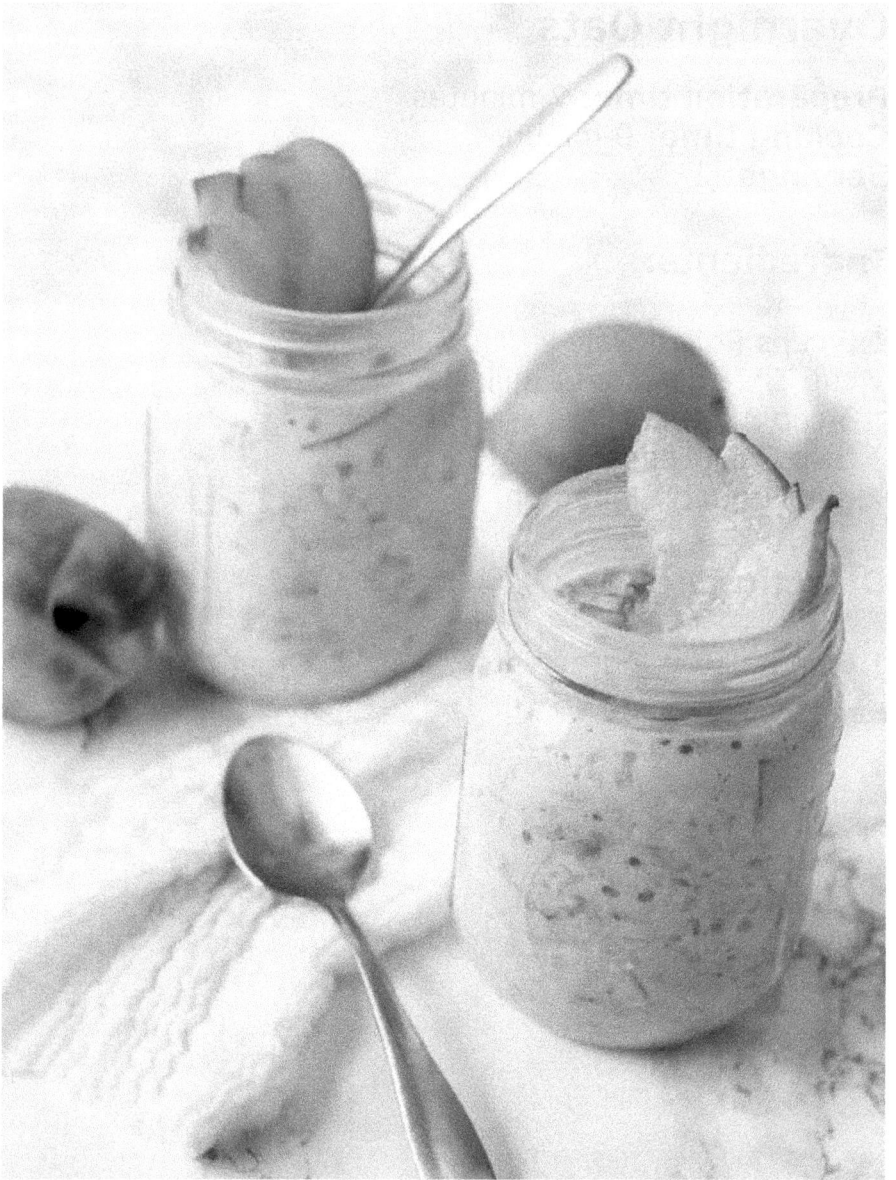

Mjadera

Preparation time: 7 minutes
Cooking time: 0 minute
Servings: 4

Ingredients:

1 Cup Brown lentils
1 cup Bulgur
1 Chopped Onion
2 tbsp Avocado or grapeseed oil
1/4 cup olive oil
Salt

Directions:

1.Wash lentils & crook in the pot along with three cups water on moderate heat for fifteen minutes. Lentils should be dente.

2.When lentils are cooking, cut the onion into dices and sauté with cooking oil and sauté and oil in a pan till brown. The darker the onion, is more flavorful the dish will be.

3.Add uncooked bulgur, caramelized onion, one-fourth cup of olive oil, 1 cup water & salt according to taste. These are added into semi- cooked lentils on moderate heat till they are cooked fully.

4.If the water dries and still lentils aren't cooked properly, add water according to need and cook again.

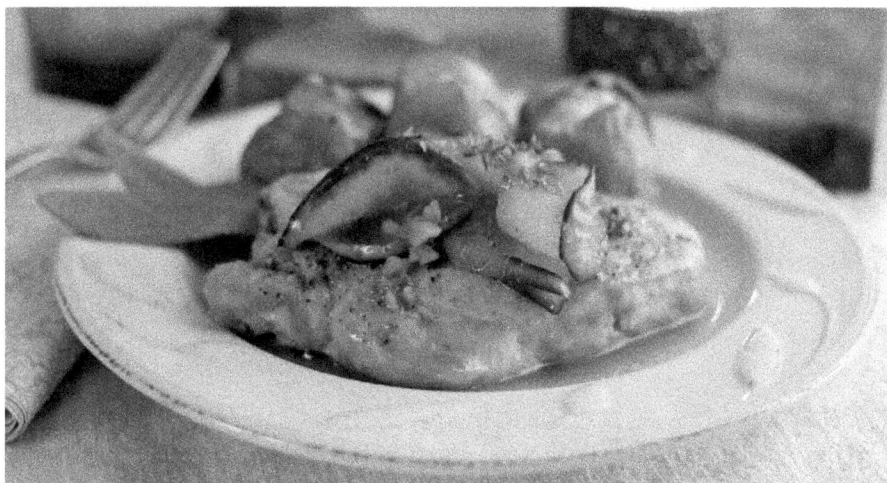

Banana Cheesecake Chocolate Cookies

Preparation Time: 20 Minutes
Cooking Time: 25 Minutes
Serving: 14 cookies

Ingredients:

Crust
2 tbsp butter
12 cookies Oreo Cheesecakes
1 tsp vanilla extract
2 tbsp flour
1/4 cup cream
1/2 cup sugar
1/2 cup chocolate chips
2 * 8 oz. cream cheese
1/2 cup banana
1 egg
Chocolate Whipped Cream
1 cup heavy whipping cream
1/4 cup cocoa powder
2 Tablespoons mini chocolate chips
1/2 cup powdered sugar
1/2 teaspoon rum extract
1 yellow banana, sliced

Directions:

1.Blend all the mixture in the blender except eggs and banana.

2. Now whisk egg and banana and make a batter.

3.Bake the batter in the oven at 350 degrees for twenty-five minutes.

4.Top the cookies with cocoa, cream, vanilla, and sugar mixture.

5.Serve and enjoy.

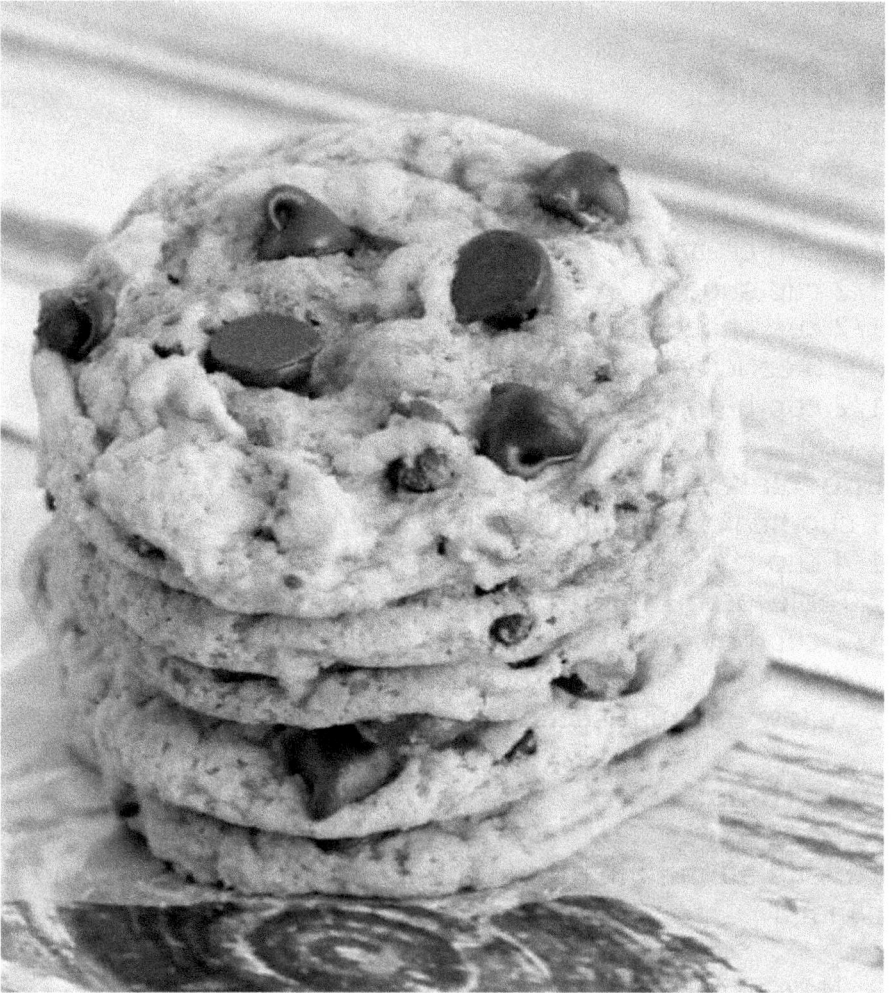

Cheesecake Ice Cream

Preparation Time: 20 Minutes
Cooking Time: 20 Minutes
Serving: 1.5 quarts

Ingredients:

1 cup milk
2 eggs
2.5 cups cream
1 tsp vanilla extract
1-1/4 cups sugar
12 oz. cream cheese
1 tbsp lemon juice

Directions:

1.Melt sugar in cream and milk mixture.

2.Whisk in egg and transfer in a pan. Cook over medium flame.

3.Remove from flame and mix in cream cheese.

4.Cool the mixture and stir in lemon juice and vanilla extract.

5.Refrigerate it for 120 minutes and serve.

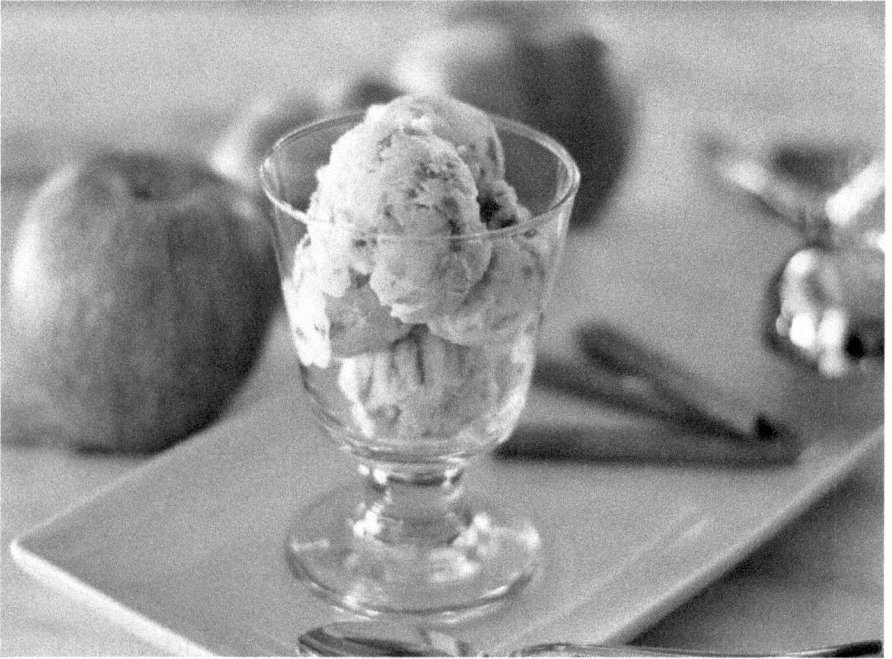

Vanilla Custard

Preparation Time: 10 minutes
Cooking Time: 20 minutes
Serving: 4

Ingredients:

1 tbsp corn-flour
1/3 cup sugar
1 Vanilla Bean
1 cup milk
4 yolks of egg
1 cup cream

Directions:

1.Cook vanilla, milk, and cream in a saucepan with continuous stirring.

2.Pour cream mixture over egg, sugar, and corn flour mixture in a bowl.

3.Cook until the required thickness is achieved.

4.Cook and serve.

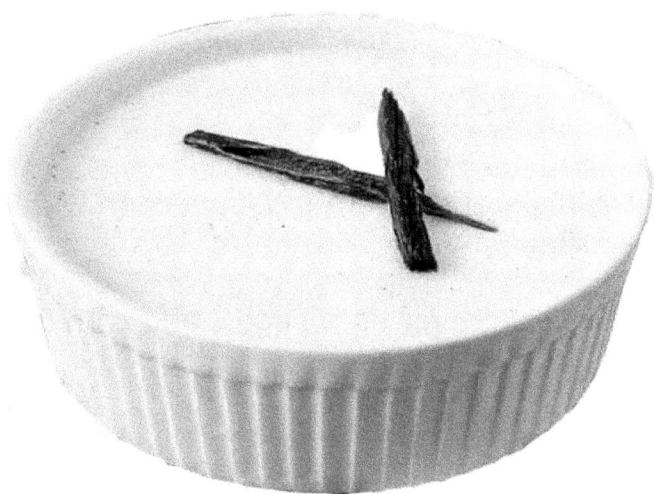

Chocolate Cheesecake Shake

Preparation Time: 10 Minutes
Cooking Time: 0 Minutes
Serving: 4

Ingredients:

6 scoops of ice cream (chocolate flavor)
8 oz. cream cheese
2 cups of milk

Directions:

1.Blend milk and cream cheese in a food processor.

2.Transfer the mixture to a serving glass and add ice cream and serve.

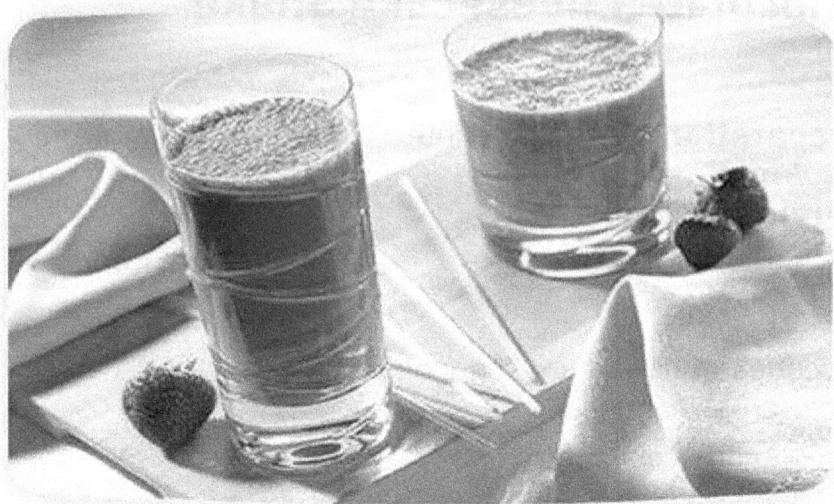

Chocolate Crunch Cookies

Preparation Time: 15 Minutes
Cooking Time: 10 Minutes
Serving: 35 cookies

Ingredients:

1/2 cups chocolate chips
1.5 cups butter
2 eggs
1 tsp baking soda
2 cups of sugar
1 tsp vanilla
One tsp salt
1/2 cup pecans
2 cups oats
2 cups flour
2 cups Krispies Rice

Directions:

1.Whisk all the ingredients in a large mixing bowl and pour the batter into a baking tray.

2.Bake in a preheated oven at 350 degrees for ten minutes.

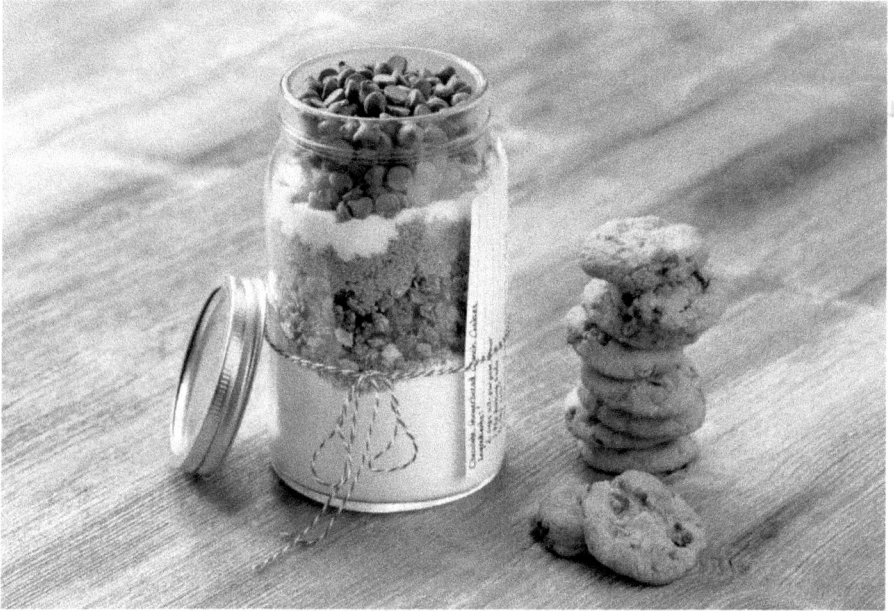

Candied Corn Puffs

Preparation Time: 15 Minutes
Cooking Time: 35 Minutes
Serving: 8

Ingredients:
8 oz corn puffs
1 cup butter
Salt as required
1 tsp baking soda
1 cup peanuts
1 cup of sugar
1.2 cup of corn syrup

Directions:

1.Boil syrup, butter, and sugar.

2. Add baking soda and transfer the mixture to a bowl with corn and peanuts.

3.Bake for 35 minutes in the oven at 250 degrees.

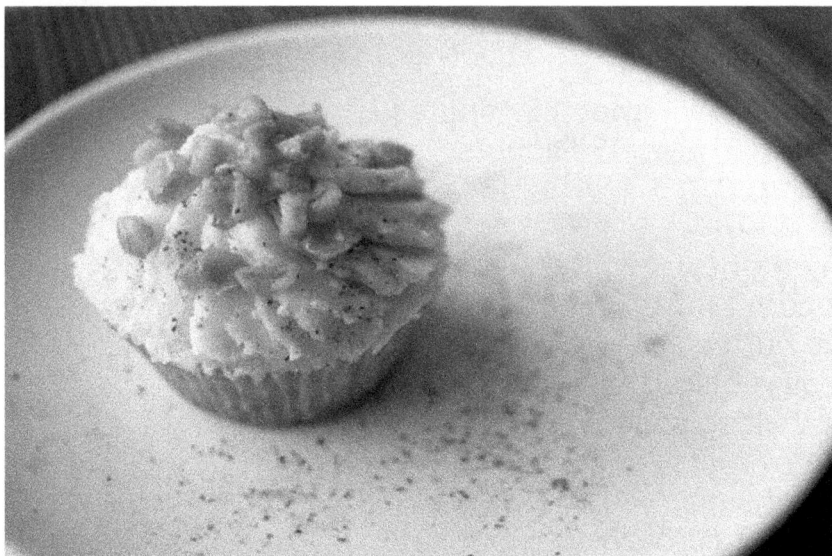

Baked cheese crisp

Preparation Time: 5 Minutes
Cooking Time: 8 Minutes
Serving: 4

Ingredients:

¾ cup shredded cheddar
¾ cup parmesan cheese
1 tsp Italian seasoning

Directions:

1.Mix cheese and place on a baking tray.

2.Bake for eight minutes in the oven at 400 degrees.

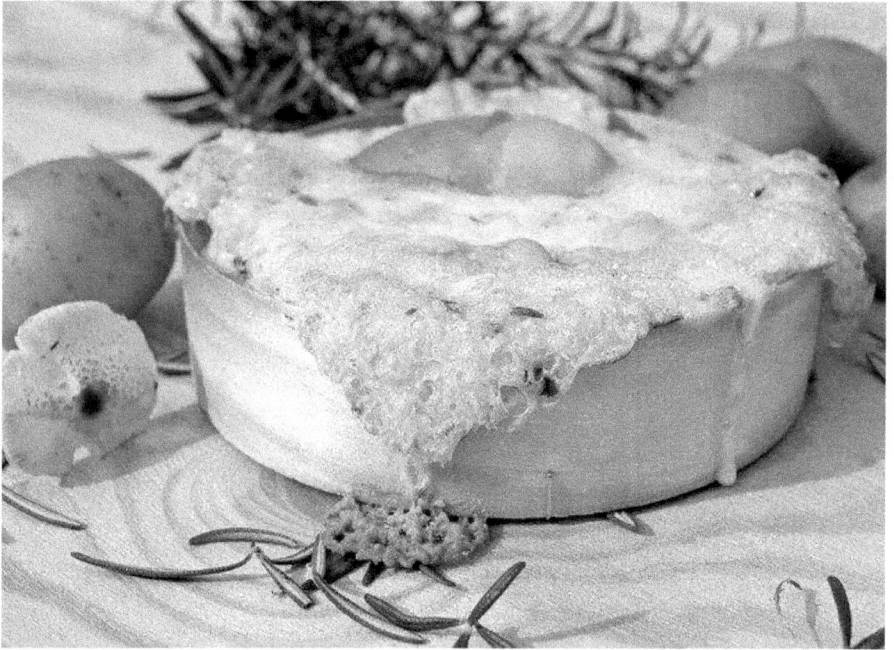

Strawberry Vinaigrette

Preparation Time: 10 minutes
Cooking time: 0 minutes
Servings: 9

Ingredients:
8 oz strawberries
Salt to taste
2 tbsp apple cider vinegar
2 tbsp honey
2 tbsp olive oil
¼ tsp black pepper

Directions:

1. Blend all the ingredients in a blender and pour in the serving dish.

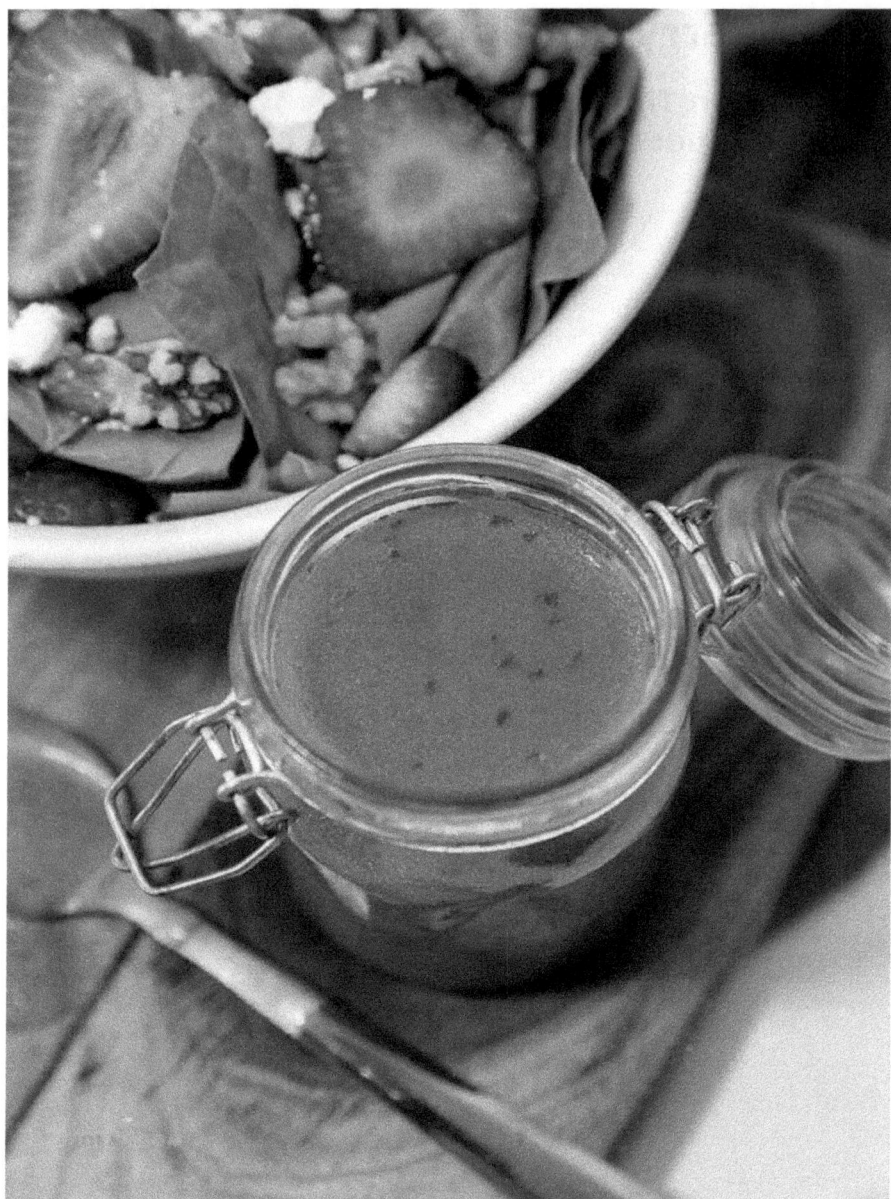

Green-Berry Smoothie

Preparation Time: 20 Minutes
Cooking Time: 0 Minutes
Servings: 2

Ingredients:

1 ripe banana
½ cup blackcurrants take off stems baby kale leaves
take off stems tsp. honey
1 cup freshly made green tea dissolve honey first in tea
then
chill
ice cubes

Directions:

1.Dissolve the honey in the tea before you relax it. Cool
first, and then blend all ingredients blender until
smooth.

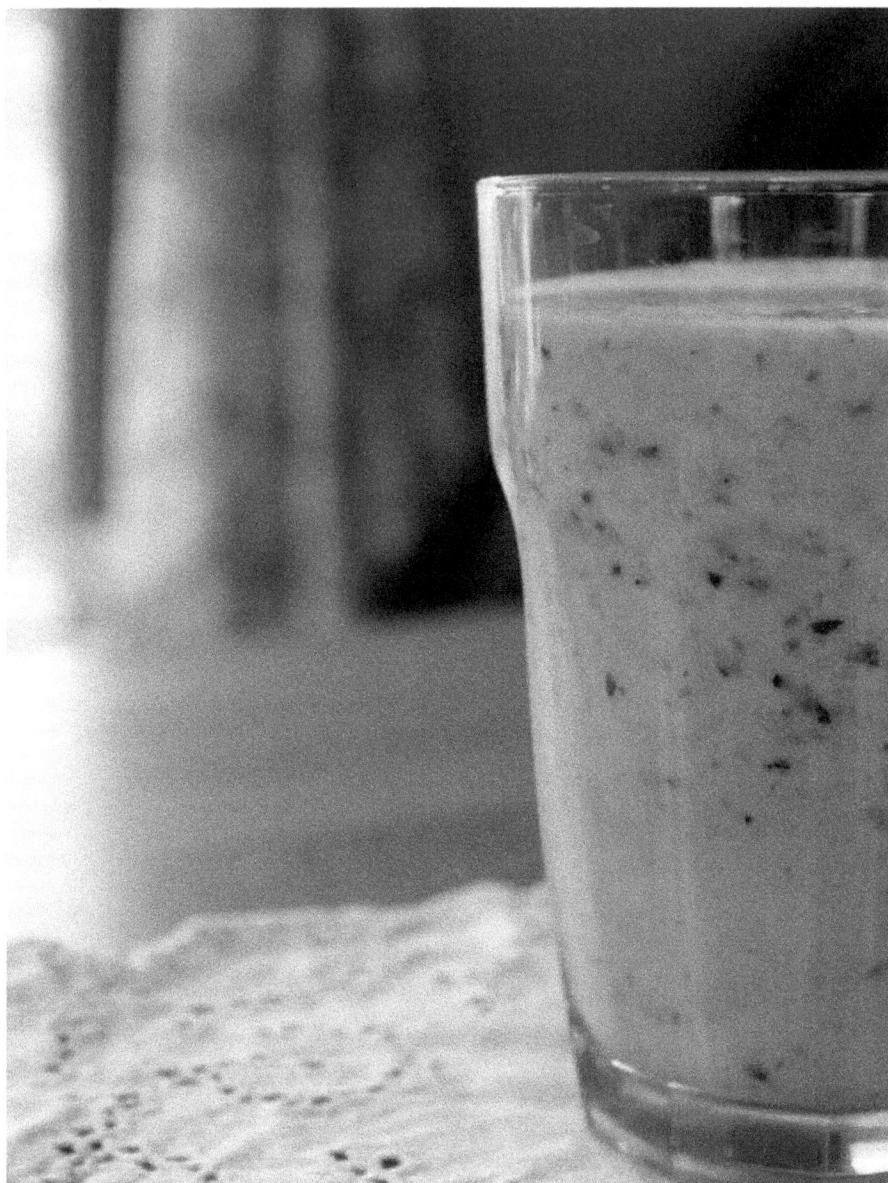

Pasta Salad Israeli

Serves:8
Preparation time: 2 hours 10 minutes
Cooking time: 10 minutes

Ingredients:

1/3 cup cucumber finely diced

1/3 cup radish diced
1/3 cup crumbled feta cheese
1/2 pound small pasta
1/3 cup tomato diced
1/3 cup yellow bell pepper diced
1/3 cup orange bell pepper diced
1/3 cup pepperoncini diced
1/3 cup black olives diced
1/3 cup green olives halved
1/3 cup red onion diced
1 tsp dried oregano
1/2 cup fresh thyme leaves
1 lemon juiced
1/4 cup olive oil more needed later on
1/2 tsp ground black pepper
1 tsp salt

Directions:

1.Place a saucepan over medium-high heat. Fill with salted water half full. Bring to boil and add your pasta. Cook this for 10 minutes until tender. After drain and rinse in cold water.

2.Transfer your pasta to a bowl add some oil and toss until fully incorporated. Add all the remaining

Ingredients: left leave the feta cheese until the end and stir well until all is mixed together.

3.Fold in cheese and refrigerate this for 2 hours. When ready to serve top the pasta salad with thyme leaves and serve.

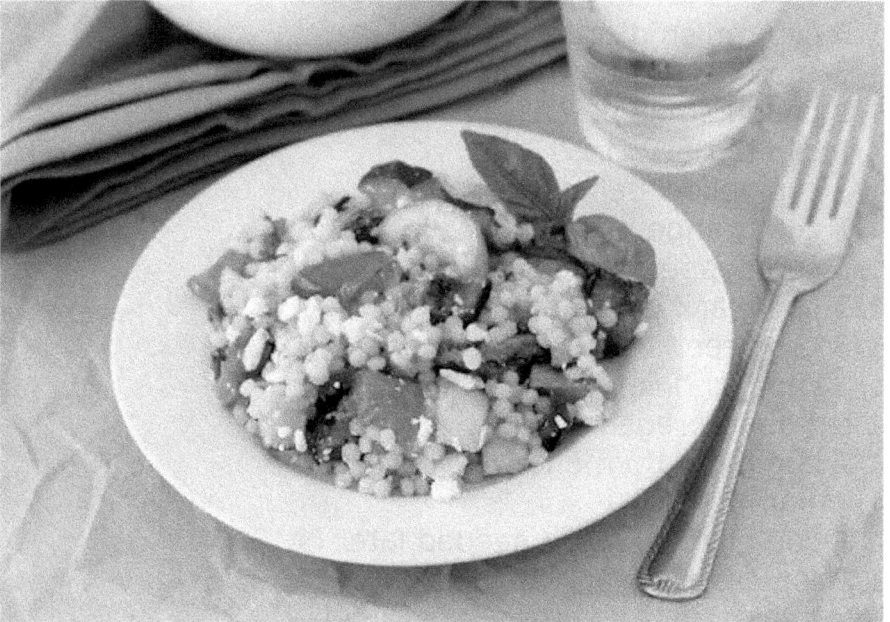

Amazing Cauliflower Pizza

Prep time cook time:1 hour 40 minutes
Servings:4

Ingredients:

The cauliflower crust:
1 1/3 cup and 4 tablespoon of grated parmesan cheese divided
3 pounds of cauliflower cut into small florets
1 tablespoon and 1 teaspoon of minced garlic
2 egg whites
1 teaspoon Italian seasoning
1/4 teaspoon of ground black pepper
1/2 teaspoon of salt
For the Greek Yogurt Basil Sauce:
1/2 cup Greek yoghurt
1/2 cup of fresh basil chopped
2 teaspoon of minced garlic
1 tablespoon of olive oil
1/2 teaspoon of salt
1/2 teaspoon of ground black pepper
For the topping:

1/2 cup of parmesan cheese grated
Roma tomatoes 3 inch 1/2 thick sliced
1 small Zucchini sliced
Fresh basil for garnish
1/2 tablespoon of olive oil
1/2 teaspoon salt
1/2 teaspoon of ground black pepper

Directions:

1.Preheat the oven to 400 degrees F. Meanwhile place a

pizza pan with parchment sheet and set it aside.

2.Next prepare the crust for this place your cauliflower florets in a food processor and pulse in batches for 1 minute until the mixture represents rice.

3.Pour riced cauliflower in a large heat proof bowl microwave that for 14 minutes make sure to stir halfway through.

4. Let the riced cauliflower stand for 15 minutes or until it is slightly cooked then wrap it into a thin towel and make sure a to twist to remove any excess moisture.

5.After that return the cauliflower into the bowl and add your black pepper salt garlic Italian seasoning and 1 1/3 cup cheese. Stir well until all have combined. Add your egg whites and mix well until incorporated. Divide the mixture into 2 balls each about 1 cup.

6.Then place onto prepared pizza pan and spread them evenly to form a nice crust and leave the ridge.

7.Place your pizza pan into the oven and bake for 30 minutes until nicely golden brown.

8.While that is baking prepare for your yoghurt basil sauce. For this blend yoghurt garlic and basil until it is creamy.

9.Blend in olive oil until it is well mixed then tip the sauce in a ball and set aside until it is needed. Now prepare the topping set grill and let preheat at medium high.

10.Place your Zucchini slices in a bowl add tomatoes and your olive oil and then season nicely with pepper and salt and toss until well coated.

11.Put these vegetables on a grill rack and cook to 3 minutes per side.

12.After it is done transfer the vegetable to a plate and set aside. Keep the grill on. When the pizza crust is cooked remove from the oven, switch on the broiler and preheat at high for 3 minutes.

13.Put 4 remains of cheese tablespoons onto the pizza crust and then place under the broiler and cook for 2 minutes until the cheese is nicely melted and brown.

14.Remove the pizza pan from oven spread yoghurt sauce on the crust and top with your grilled vegetables and cover with remaining cheese.

15.Place the pizza pan onto the grill and cook for 3 minutes until the cheese melts. Slice and serve your delicious cauliflower pizza.

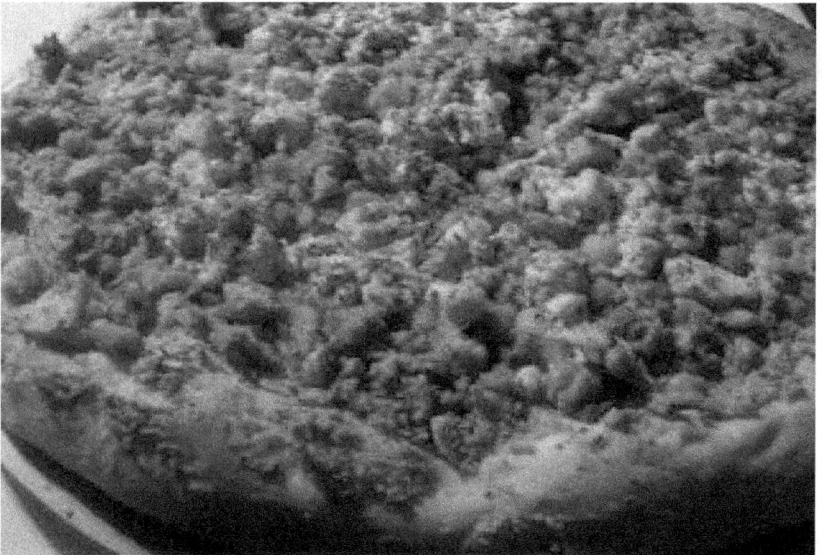

Flatbreads Mediterranean

Serves:6P
Preparation time: 10 minutes
Cooking time: 10 minutes

Ingredients:

4 ounce marinated artichoke hearts
2 cups baby spinach
1/2 cup cherry tomatoes halved
2/3 cup cannellini beans
1/2 cup medium avocado sliced
1/4 cup cherry tomatoes halved
2 ounces crumbled feta cheese
1/4 small red onion peeled and sliced
1/4 cup almond
1/8 tsp ground black pepper
1tbsp olive oil
2 tbsp water
3 pieces of pita bread
1/4 tsp for slat some extra for sprinkling

Directions:

1.Set your oven to 350 degrees F. At the same time pour beans into a food processor. Add your basil spinach salt pepper olive oil almonds and water together and pulse for 1 minute until smooth.

2.Place your flatbreads on a baking sheet and spread the bean pesto on flatbreads. Top this with your tomatoes avocado chopped artichokes and onion. Sprinkle with cheese.

3.Place your flatbread into the oven and let bake for 10 minutes or until the pita bread is lightly crispy. When done cut each pizza in slices and serve.

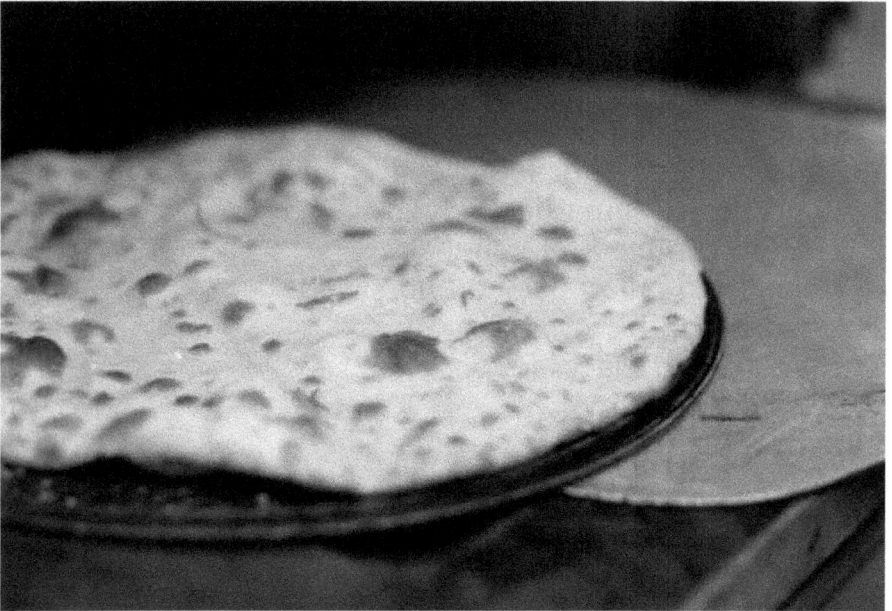

Spinach Feta Grilled Cheese

Serves: 2
Preparation time: 10 minutes
Cooking time: 18 minutes

Ingredients:
1/4 pound spinach
½ teaspoon garlic
1/8 teaspoon salt
1/8 teaspoon ground black pepper
1/8 teaspoon red pepper flakes
1/2 tablespoons olive oil
1 cup shredded mozzarella cheese
2 tablespoons crumbled feta cheese
2 ciabatta rolls halved

Directions:

1.Place a medium skillet pan over medium-low heat add oil and when hot add garlic.

2.Cook for 2 minutes or until fragrant then add spinach and stir until mixed.

3.Turn heat to medium level and cook spinach for 5 minutes or until heated through and all the cooking liquid evaporates.

4.Season with salt and black pepper and remove the pan from heat.

5.Spread ¼ cup of mozzarella cheese and 1 tablespoon feta cheese onto the bottom half of each roll top evenly with cooked spinach and then sprinkle with red pepper flakes.

6.Sprinkle with remaining mozzarella cheese and cover with top half of roll.

7.Place a large skillet pan over medium heat and place sandwiches in it.
8.Fill a large pot half full with water and place on the sandwich to press them like Panini press.

9.Switch heat to medium-low level and cook for 5 minutes or until bottom is crispy.

10.Then remove the pot flip the sandwich carefully top again with pot and continue cooking for another 5 minutes or until the other side is crispy and cheese melts completely.

11.Serve when ready.

Baba Ganoush(Vegan)

Preparation time: 10 minutes
Cook time: 15 minutes
Serves: 6

Ingredient:

1 eggplant peeled and sliced

1/4 cup tallini
1/2 teaspoon sea salt
Juice of 1 lemon
1/4 teaspoon ground cumin
1/8 teaspoon freshly ground black pepper
2 tablespoons extra-virgin olive oil
2 tablespoons sunflower seeds (optional)
2 tablespoons fresh Italian
parsley leaves (optional)

Directions:

1.Preheat the oven to 350°F.

2.Using a baking sheet spread the eggplant slices in an even layer. Bake for about 15 minutes until soft. Cool slightly and roughly chop the eggplant.

3.In a blender blend the eggplant with the tahini sea salt lemon juice cumin and pepper for about 30 seconds. Transfer to a serving dish.

4.Drizzle with the olive oil and sprinkle with the sunflower seeds and parsley (if using) before serving.

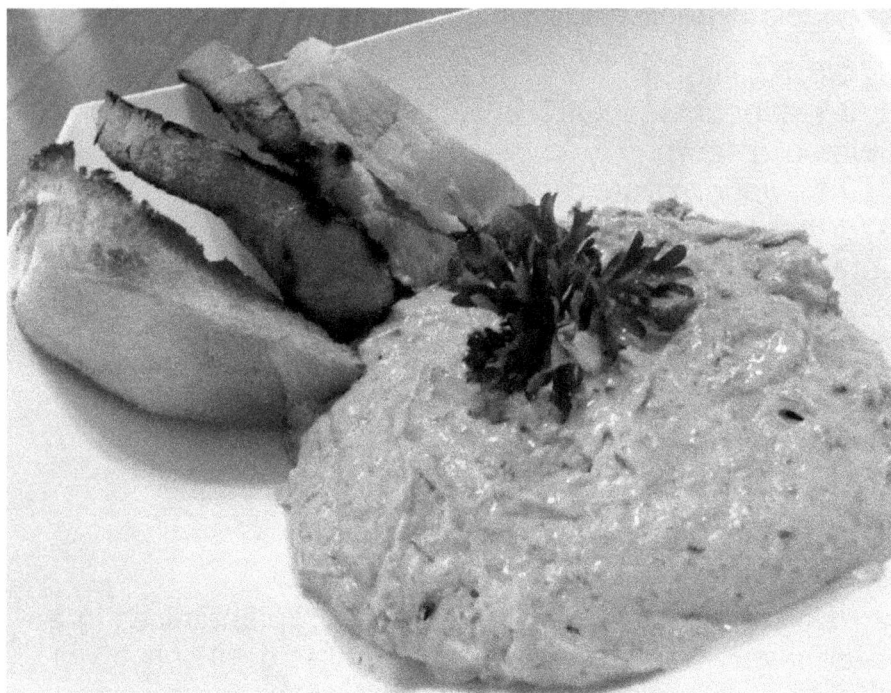

Spiced Almonds

Prep time: 10 minutes
Cook time: 7 minutes
Serves: 8

Ingredient:

2 cups raw unsalted almonds
1 tablespoon extra-virgin olive oil
1 teaspoon ground cumming
1/2 teaspoon garlic powder
1/2 teaspoon sea salt
1/8 teaspoon cayenne pepper

Directions:

1In a large nonstick skillet over medium-high heat cook the almonds for about 3 minutes shaking the pan constantly until the almonds become fragrant. Transfer to a bowl and set aside.

2.In the same skillet over medium-high heat heat the olive oil until it shimmers.
3.Add the cumin garlic powder sea salt and cayenne. Cook for 30 to 60 seconds until the spices become fragrant.

4.Add the almonds to the skillet. Cook for about 3 minutes more stirring until the spices coat the almonds.

5.Let it cool before serving.

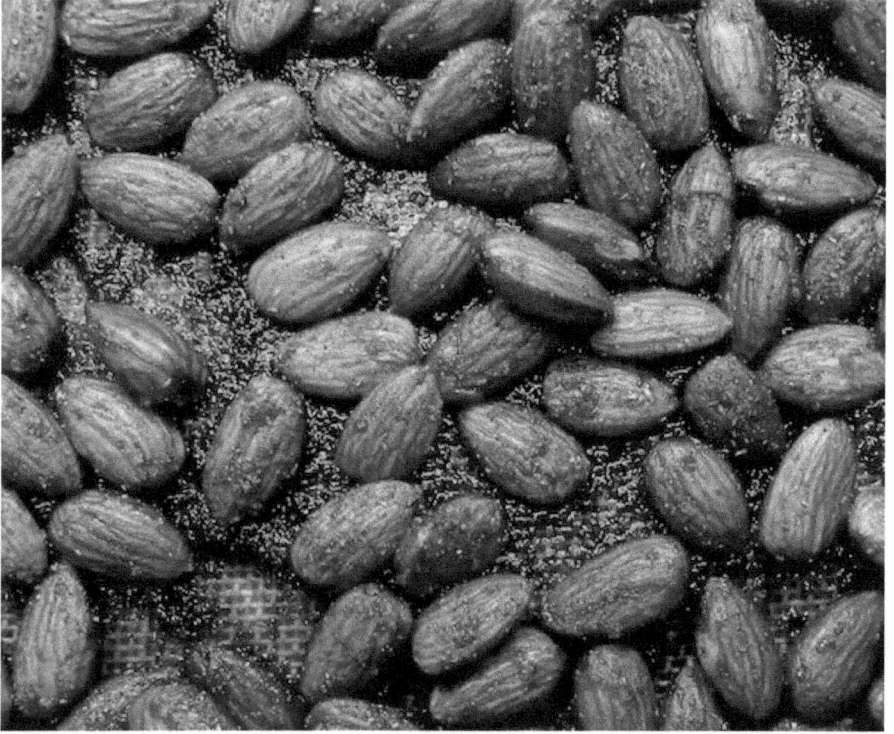

Potpourri of Plum, Pistachios & Pomegranate

Preparation Time: 30 minutes
Cooking Time: 30 minutes
Servings: 12-servings (3-cups),
Serving Size: ¼-cup

Ingredients:

Olive oil mist

1½-cups pistachios, unsalted
½-cup dried apricots, chopped
¼-cup pomegranate seeds
¼-tsp ground nutmeg
¼-tsp ground allspice
 ½-tsp cinnamon 2-tsp sugar

Directions:

1.Preheat your oven to 350 °F.

2.Spread the pistachios evenly in a rimmed baking sheet misted with olive oil. Bake for 7 minutes until lightly toasted. Let the roasted pistachios to cool completely.

3.Toss the roasted pistachios with the apricots, pomegranate seeds, nutmeg, allspice, cinnamon, and sugar until fully coated.

TIP: You can make this recipe ahead up to 3 days before eating. This dessert recipe is also ideal for solo snacks or as a topping on a cup of yogurt

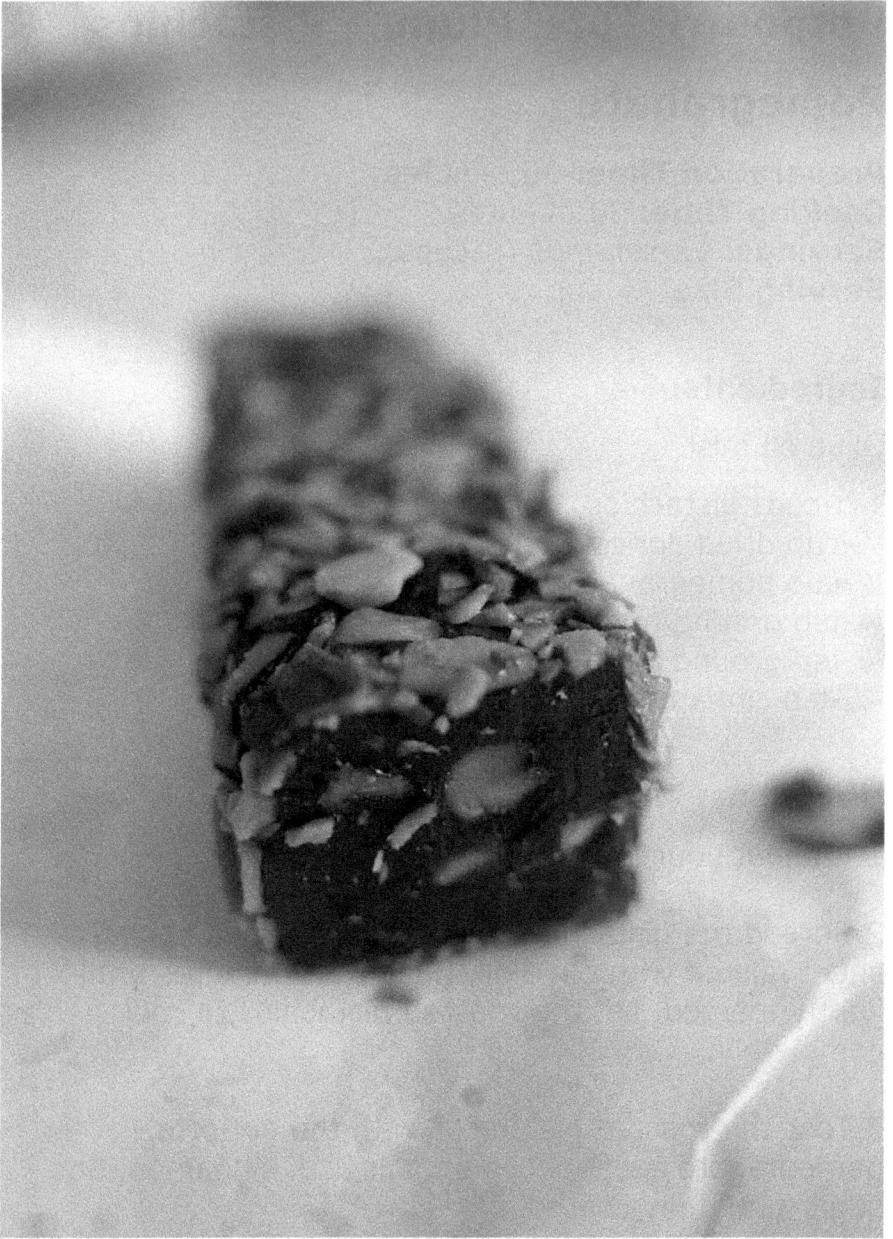

Grecian "Golden Delicious" Dessert

Preparation Time: 10 minutes
Cooking Time: 35 minutes
Servings: 8
Serving Size: 1-slice

Ingredients:

1½-lbs. Golden Delicious apples, peeled, cored, and sliced thinly (divided)
1- pcs eggs
Zest of lemon, grated
⅓ -cup brown sugar A pinch of salt
¼-cup plus 1-tbsp low-fat milk 3-tsp baking powder
1 cup less 1-tbsp whole-wheat flour, sifted
1-tbsp light brown sugar for topping (optional)
1-tbsp icing sugar for dusting

Directions:

1.Preheat your oven to 350 °F. Prepare a greased and flour-sprinkled 8" x 8" baking pan. Set aside.

2.Combine and mix the eggs, lemon zest, sugar, and salt in your stand mixer's mixing bowl. Beat to a creamy and thick consistency.

3.Pour in the milk, and add the baking powder and flour. Beat until fully incorporated.

4.Add ⅔ or 1-pound of the sliced apples to the batter. By using a spatula, mix thoroughly until fully combined. Transfer the batter in the prepared baking pan.

5.Top the batter with the remaining apple slices. If desired, sprinkle with a tablespoon of brown sugar.

6.Place the pan in the preheated oven. Bake for 35 minutes until an inserted toothpick into the center of the apple cake comes out clean.

7.To serve, dust the low-fat cake with icing sugar.

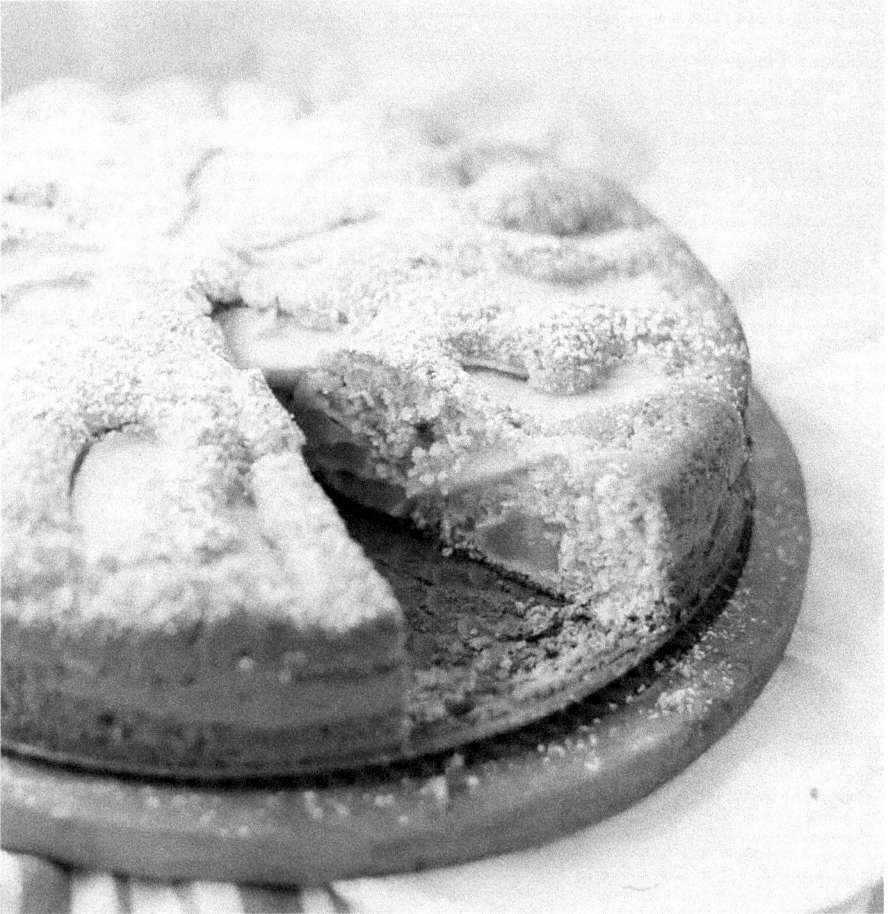

Chocolate Covered Strawberries

Preparation time: 15 Minutes
Servings: 24 servings

Ingredients:

16 ounces milk chocolate chips
2 tablespoons shortening
1-pound fresh strawberries with leaves

Directions:
1.In a bain-marie, melt chocolate and shorter, occasionally stirring until smooth. Hold them by the toothpicks and immerse the strawberries in the chocolate mixture.

2.Put toothpicks in the top of the strawberries.

3.Turn the strawberries and put the toothpick in the styrofoam so that the chocolate cools.

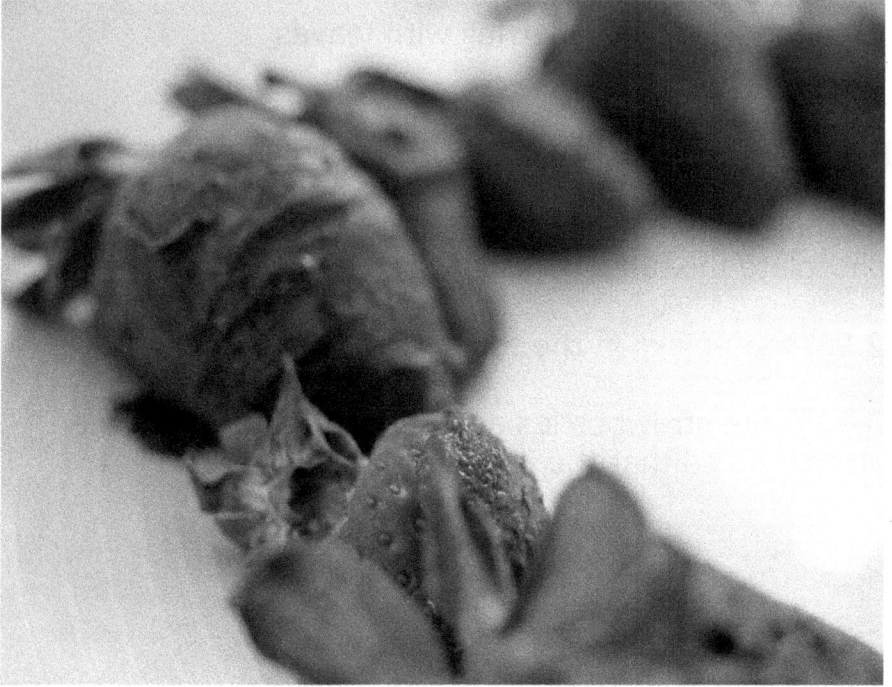

Strawberry Angel Food Dessert

Preparation time: 15 minutes
Servings: 18 servings

Ingredients:

1 angel cake (10 inches)
2 packages of softened cream cheese
1 cup of white sugar
1 container (8 oz) of frozen fluff, thawed
1 liter of fresh strawberries, sliced
1 jar of strawberry icing

Directions:

1.Crumble the cake in a 9 x 13-inch dish.

2.Beat the cream cheese and sugar in a medium bowl until the mixture is light and fluffy. Stir in the whipped topping. Crush the cake with your hands, and spread the cream cheese mixture over the cake.

3.Combine the strawberries and the frosting in a bowl until the strawberries are well covered. Spread over the layer of cream cheese.

4.Cool until ready to serve.

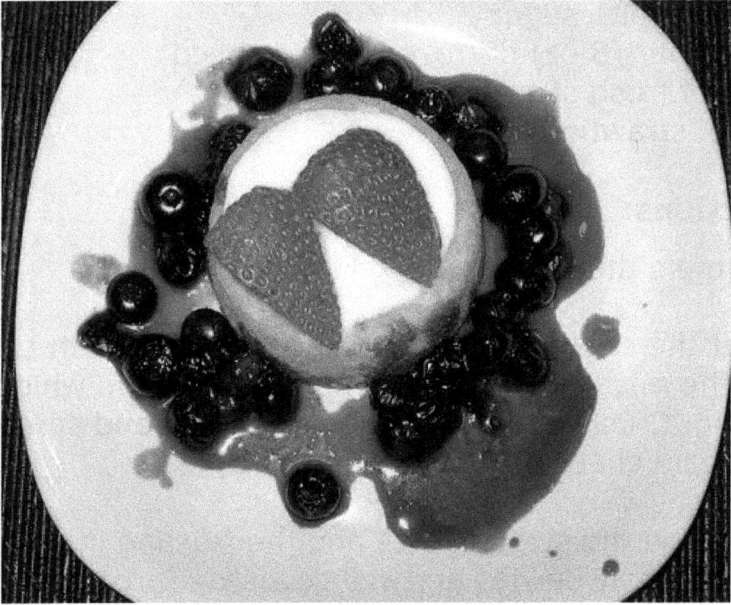

Fruit Pizza

Preparation time: 30 Minutes
Servings: 8 servings

Ingredients:

Sugar cookie dough in a cooled package of 1 oz (18 oz),

cream cheese in a package of 1 (8 ounces), softened

1 (8 oz.) Frozen defrosted filling, defrosted
2 cups of freshly cut strawberries
1/2 cup of white sugar, 1 pinch of salt
1 tablespoon corn flour
2 tablespoons lemon juice
1/2 cup orange juice
1/4 cup water
1/2 teaspoon orange zest

Directions:

1.Preheat the oven to 175 ° C (350 ° F). Slice the cookie dough then place it on a greased pizza pan. Press the dough flat into the mold. 2.Bake for 10 to 12 minutes. Let cool.

2.Soften the cream cheese in a large bowl and then stir in the whipped topping. Spread over the cooled crust. You can relax for a moment at this stage or continue to arrange the fruit.

3.Start with strawberries cut in half. Place them in a circle around the outer edge. Continue with the fruit of your choice by going to the center. If you use bananas, immerse them in lemon juice so that they do not get dark. Then make a sauce with a spoon on the fruit.

4.Combine sugar, salt, corn flour, orange juice, lemon juice, and water in a pan. Boil and stir over medium heat. Bring to the boil and cook for 1 or 2 minutes until thick. Remove from heat and add the grated orange zest. Cool, but not in place. Place on the fruit.

5.Allow to cool for two hours, cut into quarters, and serve.

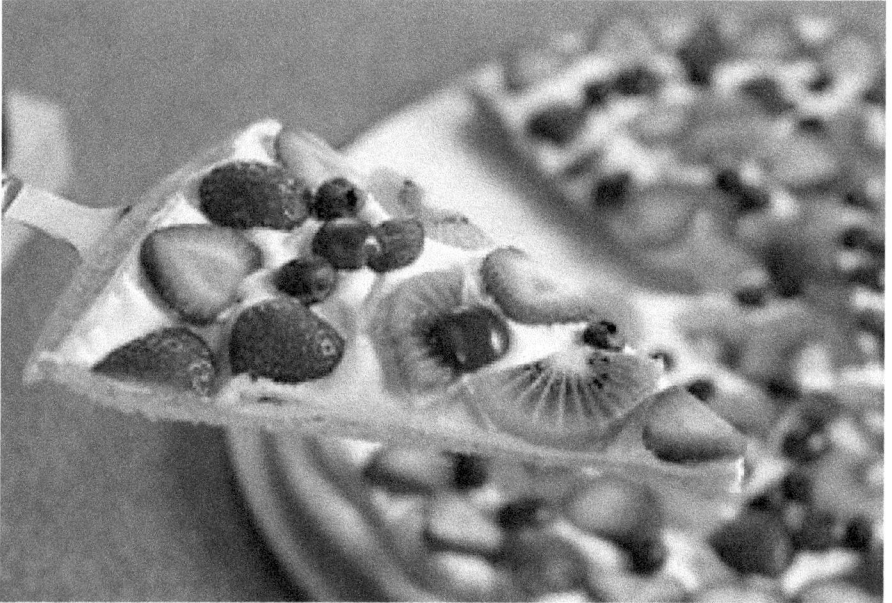

Bananas Foster

Preparation time: 5 minutes
Servings: 4 Servings

Ingredients:

2/3 cup dark brown sugar
1/4 cup butter
3 1/2 tablespoons rum
1 1/2 teaspoon vanilla extract
1/2 teaspoon of ground cinnamon
3 bananas, peeled and cut lengthwise and broad
¼ cup coarsely chopped nuts1, vanilla ice cream

Directions:

1.Melt the butter in a big, deep frying pan over medium heat. Stir in sugar, rum, vanilla, and cinnamon.

2.When the mixture starts to bubble, place the bananas and nuts in the pan. Bake until the bananas are hot, 1 to 2 minutes.

3.Serve immediately on a vanilla ice cream.

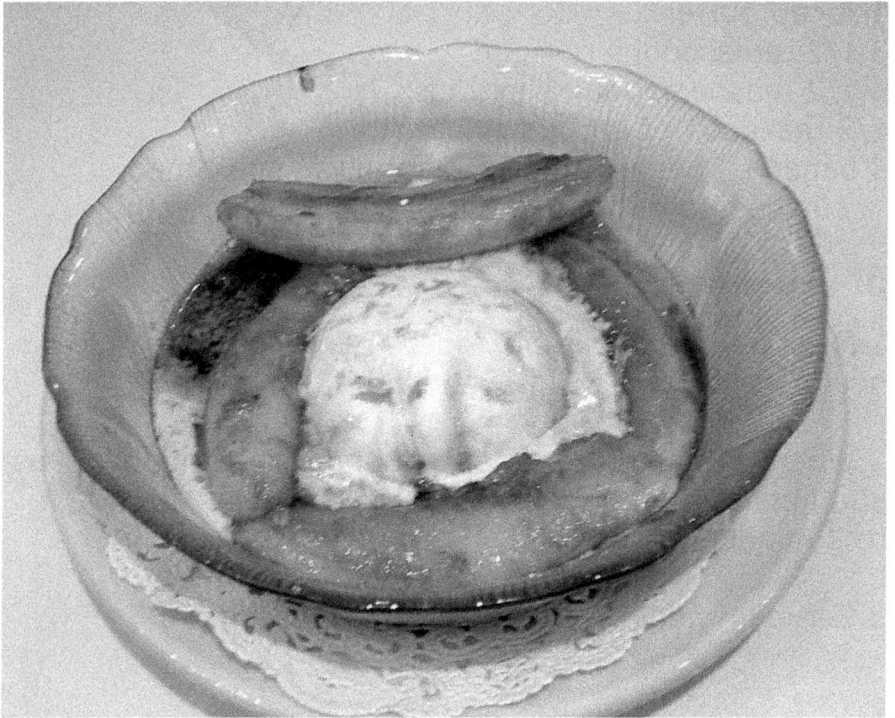

Cranberry Orange Cookies

Preparation time: 20 Minutes
Servings: 48 servings

Ingredients:
1 cup of soft butter
1 cup of white sugar
1/2 cup brown sugar
1 egg
1 teaspoon grated orange peel
2 tablespoons orange juice
2 1/2 cups flour, 1/2 teaspoon baking powder
1/2 teaspoon salt
2 cups chopped cranberries
1/2 cup chopped walnuts (optional)
1/2 teaspoon grated orange peel
3 tablespoons orange juice
1 ½ cup confectioner's sugar

Direction:

1.Preheat the oven to 190 ° C.
Combine butter, white sugar, and brown sugar in a large bowl until smooth.

2.Beat the egg until everything is well mixed. Mix 1 teaspoon of orange zest and 2 tablespoons of orange juice. Mix the flour, baking powder, and salt; stir in the orange mixture. Mix the cranberries and, if used, the nuts until well distributed. Place the dough per rounded soup spoon on ungreased baking trays. The cookies must be placed at least 2 inches away.

3.Bake in the preheated oven for 12 to 14 minutes, until the edges are golden brown. Remove baking trays to cool on racks.

4.Get a small bowl, mix 1/2 teaspoon of orange peel, 3 tablespoons of orange juice, and icing confectionery ingredients. Spread over cooled cookies. Let's act

Key Pie Vill

Preparation time: 15 minutes
Servings: 8 Servings

Ingredients:

1 (9 inches) prepared graham cracker crust 3 cups of
sweetened condensed milk
1/2 cup sour cream 3/4 cup lime juice
1 tablespoon grated lime zest

Directions:

1.Preheat the oven to 175 ° C (350 ° F).
Combine the condensed milk, sour cream, lime juice,
and lime zest in a medium bowl. Mix well and pour into
the graham cracker crust.

2.Bake in the preheated oven for 5 to 8 minutes until
small hole bubbles burst on the surface of the cake.
DON'T BROWN! Cool the cake well before serving.
Decorate with lime slices and whipped cream if desired.

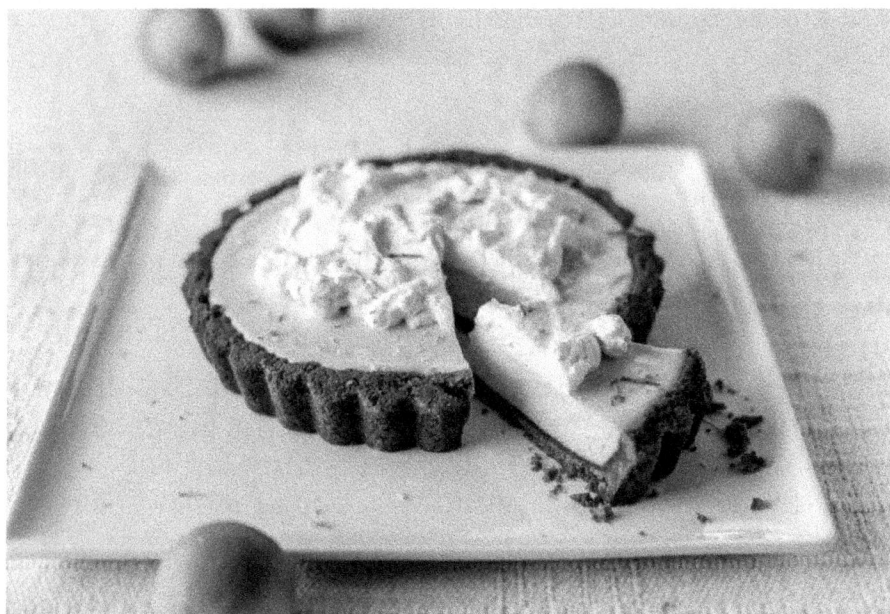

Sweet Popcorn

Prep time: 5 minutes
Cook time: 15 minutes
Serve 8

Ingredient:

8 cups air-popped popcorn

2 tablespoons extra-virgin olive oil
2 tablespoons packed brown sugar
2 tablespoons Chinese five-spice powder
1/4 teaspoon sea salt

Directions:

1.Preheat the oven to 350°F.

2.Put the popcorn in a large bowl. Set aside.

3.In a small bowl whisk the olive oil brown sugar five-spice powder and sea salt. Pour the mixture over the popcorn tossing to coat. Transfer to a 9-by- 13-inch baking dish.

4.Bake the popcorn for 15 minutes stirring every 5 minutes or so. Serve hot or cool and store in resealable bags in single-serve (1-cup) batches.

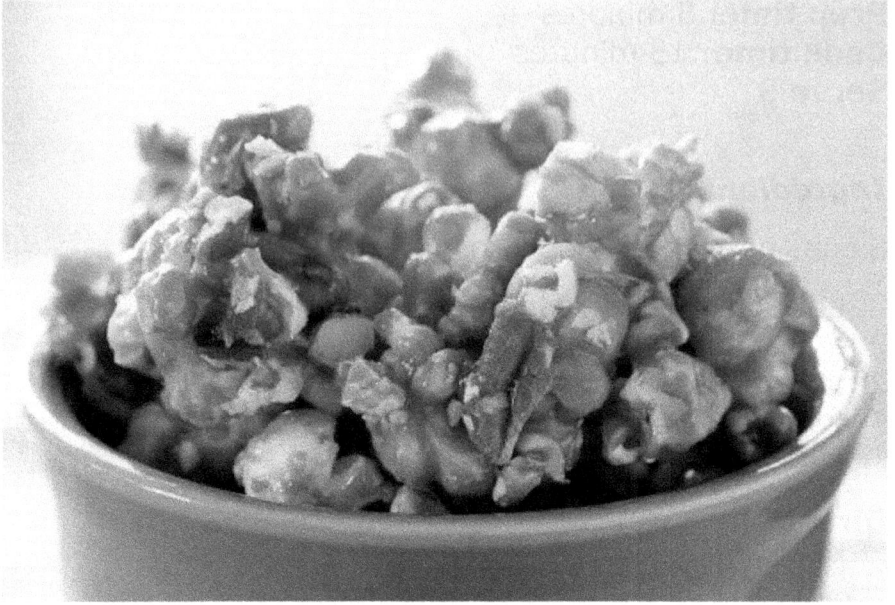